ISCADOR

Iscador Facts

- Iscador is a prescription medicine in injectable form developed in Europe.
- It has been in continuous use since 1917.
- It is the cancer drug most recognized by name in Germany.
- Over sixty percent of cancer patients in Germany use some form of mistletoe.
- Iscador is more often prescribed by oncologists and conventional physicians than by complementary physicians.
- Millions of doses of Iscador are sold worldwide each year.
- Iscador is a Class-P homeopathic tincture of *viscum album* diluted to a clinically safe dosage.
- Over 100 studies have been done on Iscador.

ISCADOR

Mistletoe and Cancer Therapy

Christine Murphy, Editor

Panacea Wellness Guide

Lantern Books • New York
A Division of Booklight Inc.

2001
Lantern Books
One Union Square West, Suite 201
New York, NY 10003

Printed in the United States of America

Library of Congress Cataloging-in-Publication Data

Iscador : mistletoe and cancer therapy / Christine Murphy, editor.
    p. cm.
Includes bibliographical references.
ISBN 1-930051-76-X
    1. European mistletoe—Therapeutic use. 2. Cancer—Alternative treatment. I. Murphy, Christine.

RC271.M5 I83 2001
616.99'406—dc21

2001029962

Cellular pathology and cellular physiology are under a misconception when they designate the cell as the basis of all life and regard the human organism merely as a conglomeration of cells. The truth is that the human being is to be seen as a totality, in relation to the cosmos, and constantly battling with the separate being of the cells. In reality, it is the cell which constantly disturbs our organism instead of building it up.

It is in the nature of the cell to maintain a separate existence. It must constantly be modified and differentiated to perform the organism's tasks and goals. By serving the organism, the cell must sacrifice its own separate existence. Only then will it become a true organ cell.

It is not the cells in their growth which regulate the functions of the organism but rather the organism which takes hold of the cells and designates their functions. What regulates or determines the cell in relationship to the organism lies beyond the cell. When an ovum is fertilized it subdivides inwardly at first without increasing in size. Such a cell is primitive and must learn to differentiate itself. This is learned from outside, from the forces of form and growth which are impressed into it.

—Friedrich Lorenz, MD,
from *Cancer: A Mandate To Humanity*

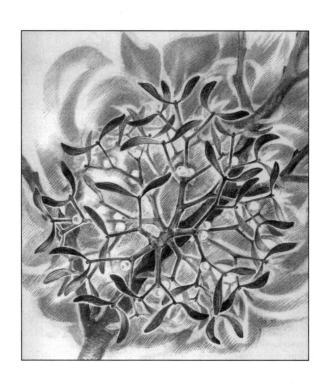

Acknowledgments

PROFOUND GRATITUDE TO THE MANY CON-tributors to this book. Among them, in particular: For the ideas: Rudolf Steiner (1861–1925), the modern ren-aissance philosopher and scientist who, early last century, sug-gested to medical doctors injections of mistletoe extract for cancer treatment. His recommendations were first put to clini-cal use by Ita Wegman, MD, and later used and developed by an ever growing number of physicians worldwide.

For the research: Since 1935 the Society of Cancer Research (Hiscia) in Arlesheim, Switzerland, has been concentrating its efforts on the manufacture, research, and development of Iscador.

For treatments in a caring atmosphere: The Lukas Clinic in Arlesheim, Switzerland, is an efficient hospital in a truly healing setting specializing in cancer treatment with Iscador.

For providing the product and literature: The Weleda Company, located in Switzerland next to Hiscia and the Lukas Clinic widely distributes Iscador and a full range of homeo-pathic/ anthroposophical remedies and body care preparations. Iscador, or Iscar as it is known in the United States, is available from Weleda, Inc., in Congers, New York.

For pioneering education of the anthroposophical approach to health and illness including Iscador: Drs. Rita Leroi and Walther Buehler. Practicing physicians, Dr. Leroi ran the Lukas Clinic for many years and Dr. Buehler created a patient organ-ization, Verein für Anthroposophisches Heilwesen, in Germany and Switzerland.

For compiling research and development: Thomas Schuerholz, MD, and David Riley, MD.

For his stature and success as an oncologist using Iscador and the anthroposophical approach: Richard Wagner, MD.

For providing courage: Authors Cheryl Sanders and Robert Sardello, directors of the School for Spiritual Psychology in Greensboro, NC.

For practical self-help tips: Dr. Erika Merz from the Helixor Company.

For art therapy: Phoebe Alexander, head of the Association for Anthroposophical Art Therapy in North America, and for nutrition: Louise Frazier.

For the use of Dr. Wagner's text, Mercury Press.

For his translations: Harold Jurgens.

For inspired editing: Gerald Karnow, M.D., Grace Ann Starkey, Michele Sanz-Cardona, Liz Pentin, and Joanna Berkowitz.

For his artistic renderings of the mistletoe plant, Walther Roggenkamp.

For speedy and supportive publishing: Lantern Books.

Thank you all, and thank you to those others who also provided help.

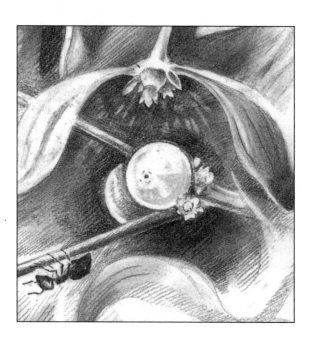

Table of Contents

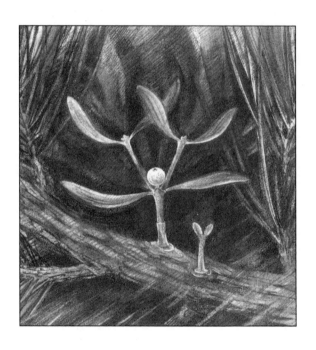

Preface

Christine Murphy

RECENTLY ISCADOR, THE MISTLETOE CANCER preparation used as an adjunct in cancer therapy, has been very much in the news. Yet it is not a new medicine. Once, three quarters of a century ago, Iscador was practically unknown in Europe. Since then, without promotion but with ongoing scientific investigation and refinement, it has become the most widely recognized mistletoe cancer medicine in Switzerland and Germany.

In Switzerland and Germany sixty percent of all cancer patients are now prescribed mistletoe at some point in their treatment. Many receive it for weeks before surgery and most take it for years afterwards to help prevent recurrence. The test of time is also a test.

Iscador is an integral element of a wholistic treatment method called the anthroposophical approach to health and

illness. This method addresses body, soul, and spirit of the
patient, recognizing that every illness bears within it the seeds
of change and the possibility for new direction. It includes full
acceptance of proven scientific methods as well as homeopathy,
anthroposophical medicine, phytotherapy, art therapy, massage,
counseling and more.

The personal involvement of the physician towards attain-
ing wellness is central to the anthroposophical approach, as is
the understanding that we are responsible for our own destiny
and that illness is not a random shot fired at us from outside.
The doctor need not be conversant in the anthroposophical
approach to prescribe Iscador, but the approach adds a much
greater dimension to therapy in general.

This book is written in clear and understandable language
so that you, reading it, can come to your own informed conclusions. It describes conventional treatments and terminology
and other complementary therapies, of which Iscador is a part.
Every previously unknown medicine and method has been
subject to ridicule or destructive criticism, often by people or
groups who have no direct experience of it. This book makes no
claim to miracles. But it does outline a new look at cancer, and
as such we hope it will give you comfort and encouragement.
After all, mistletoe is the symbol of warmth and love.

The articles, some condensed from the journal LILIPOH,
and the resources at the end should enable you take your
inquiries further, helping to clarify your own choices and
wishes.

Foreword
Spiritual Courage and Illness

Cheryl Sanders and Robert Sardello

A SEVENTY-YEAR OLD MAN, FULL OF LIFE AND energy and interest in everything around him came to a doctor because he was passing blood in his urine. He felt well and had never been seriously ill before.

A physical examination revealed that the man's right kidney was enlarged. These two symptoms, along with the patient's age strongly suggested that there was a malignant tumor on the right kidney.

In order to confirm this diagnosis the doctor told this man he would have to go to the hospital for further tests. The tests confirmed a growth. The doctor now told the man that the ailment was most likely very serious. If the tumor was malignant the kidney would have to be removed and other treatments prescribed to try and prevent the spread of the cancer. The doctor then told him the possible consequences of not operating. If he did have a malignant tumor, it would quickly spread to the other kidney. He would almost certainly suffer a great deal.

This sequence of events, a sequence that happens thousands of times each day, prompts us to consider the necessity of spiritual courage in meeting the pronouncement of a disease such as cancer. Indeed, the very existence of this disease and its prevalence in the world calls us to develop the virtue of spiritual courage as an ongoing aspect of our lives. The virtue of courage is not a quality that just comes forward at times of extreme need or duress. We have to take the notion of courage and extend it into the very manner in which we live from moment to moment. What then, is spiritual courage?

Spiritual courage consists of the inner capacity to face fear without being overwhelmed by it, not due to having any personal power, but actually, through completely relinquishing any personal power whatsoever. Spiritual courage, then, differs from what we would ordinarily consider an *act* of courage. It may be courageous to immediately opt for surgery, chemotherapy, and extended treatment when one is diagnosed with cancer, or it may be courageous to explore all the possible alternatives. Spiritual courage, however, requires relinquishing the tendency toward an immediate heroic response, and instead opening oneself with all possible effort to the spiritual realms, deepening into the soul realm, and developing an intense inner listening.

In our time, a false flight from illness, nurtured by the strictly modern and materialistic fantasy that a technical

approach to medicine can restore health, has effectively eliminated the imagination of illness as bearing value. Even alternative medicine is caught in the imagination of health as the norm
and illness as a senseless deviation. Inner listening is required to
include the soul and spirit in a true process of healing. Illness,
approached with inner listening, makes us aware of the fullness
of our being, assists us in becoming aware of how we may have
become forgetful of the subtle dimensions of inner life, callous
toward the beauty of the world, habitual in our response to
others. It can make us aware that the ravages of the body cannot
touch the eternal individuality of our spirit.

In times of strong fear, bound to occur with a life-threatening illness, particular and caring attention must be given to the
soul and spirit. Otherwise, dissociation from the truth and
ground of our being occurs as we turn ourselves over to treatment systems which tend to be abstract. The greatest degree of
concentration and attentiveness is needed if we are to not just
endure the illness but seek to understand the part it has to play
in our individual destiny.

The great challenge of serious illness is more than finding
the way to stay alive; the challenge is to remain *intensely* alive,
see the spiritual significance in all things, even illness, and all
the while responding to the moment and the qualities that
accompany it.

This challenge sounds like an awesome task, one very hard
to imagine as possible without preparation taken place long
before the onset of the illness. Development of spiritual courage
requires attuning our thoughts to spiritual realities in a regular
and ongoing manner. This does not mean merely thinking

about God, the angels, Christ, or those who have died. That kind of thinking alone can never develop spiritual courage. An apt way to describe spiritual thinking is with the term "inner clarity."

With such a term, we have something deeper in mind than absence of confusion, or good logic. Inner clarity means concentrating, contemplating, meditating on the inner significance of the beings and actions of the spiritual realm to the point that these realities become luminous from within. This kind of activity develops the virtue of spiritual courage. With spiritual courage we can go through illness with a true and abiding sense of individuality of soul and spirit, even if we must undergo the humiliation of treatments which tend to treat us as abstractions rather than individual human beings.

With spiritual courage we no longer act out of personal desires, motives, urges, impulses, and ideas, but rather allow ourselves to be vessels through which spirit works through us fully consciously. Through the practical spirituality of courage we develop a kind of double-vision. The ordinary realm of perception, feeling, thinking, and action goes on, but everything in these modes of experience is also seen as corresponding to something of a spiritual nature. This spiritual intensification of life can see us through the most difficult trials imaginable.

When the doctor told the man spoken of above that he would have to go to the hospital, the man refused. He wanted to stay at home. The doctor asked the man to consider those around him—his wife, his children, his friends. What was the use in staying home and dying instead of having the disease treated and at least gaining more time. The man still refused.

He did not intend to just go home and wait, but would take care of himself in the most natural ways possible. Something of an inner nature told this person that if he allowed himself to be put into the alien world of the hospital he would lose the inner sense of who he was.

We may not agree with the decision of this individual. It does not matter. We have to admire him. Somewhere, from deep within, he knew that to be taken to the hospital, dressed in a drafty gown, put into a room with strangers, poked and probed by doctors, would mean that he would never again belong to himself. He knew in his very soul that he would never recover from the separation from himself. For others, submitting to the treatment would be right. For still others the exploration of complementary treatments would be right. This story is important, not because of the content of what the person did, but because this person approached illness out of his true individuality.

Cheryl Sanders and Robert Sardello *are Co-directors of the School of Spiritual Psychology. The School offers courses throughout the country and a two year training in sacred service. For information: PO Box 5099, Greensboro, NC 27435, phone: (336) 279-8259.*

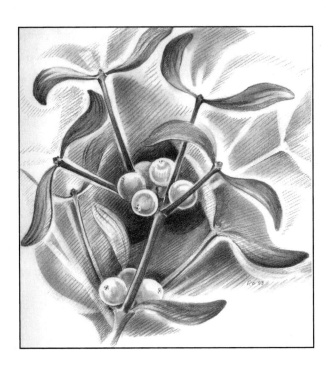

Integrative Cancer Treatment:
A Guide for Patients and Their Families

Thomas Schuerholz, MD

In 1996 an American by the name of Lance Armstrong lay in a hospital with metastasizing testicular cancer. In July 1999 the same man won the Tour de France, the toughest bicycle race on earth. This is an encouraging example, don't you agree?

THE FOLLOWING GUIDELINES ARE MEANT for all those affected by cancer: people who know they have cancer—maybe they've just found out, maybe they've been living with it for years; people waiting for the results of cancer tests; or people for whom cancer has become a real issue because a friend or relative has recently been diagnosed with the disease.

Cancer is a vital issue in the literal sense of the word. Countless experts have dealt with it from all aspects, and new findings arise almost daily. Some of this knowledge should be available to you, as a person directly or indirectly involved. Many important decisions are to be made during the course of this illness, and doctors aren't the only ones to make them.

How can we decide on a method of treatment that best fits a particular cancer; one that offers the most promising results? Doctors can be familiar with various approaches, but often it is the patient, or his or her family, who can best decide what may be most suitable—based on strengths, weaknesses, likes and dislikes.

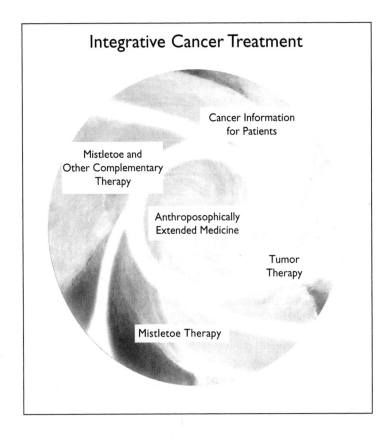

Integrative Cancer Treatment

Cancer Information for Patients

Mistletoe and Other Complementary Therapy

Anthroposophically Extended Medicine

Tumor Therapy

Mistletoe Therapy

In this chapter we will survey the types and causes of cancer, as well as usual treatment measures used today. We will also outline a number of concepts underlying integrative cancer treatment, of which mistletoe therapy plays an important part. "Integrative" means to bring all reasonable available therapeutic measures to bear on the cancer, treating it from as many sides as possible.

When you finish reading this outline, you will know more about cancer and its treatment, and be better able to talk with doctors, and make decisions about therapy.

Whether you are affected by cancer directly or indirectly— we wish with our whole heart that the treatments you choose will lead to success and renewed health.

Cancer: A Biological Process We Live With

At the beginning of the last century cancer was the seventh largest cause of death. Today it is the second, and it is estimated that by the year 2005 it will be the primary cause of death worldwide.

Although cancer specialists (oncologists) around the globe have tried for decades to cure cancer, they have yet to succeed. Only the patients themselves can overcome this illness and, depending on individual circumstances, the prospects are often good. Some patients have survived even when things looked statistically hopeless. That is why it is important to consider each case by itself, and to treat it individually.

Many people die each year from cancer and many more are newly diagnosed. Yet each one, in addition to being part of a statistic, is also an individual case.

Being diagnosed with cancer may mean many things, not simply having a sickness. It could also mean the intervention of destiny, a chance, a biographical turning point, a real-life drama, or a tragedy. But cancer is always a biological process that belongs to *life*. How is this so?

How Cancer Arises

Millions of cells die in our body every day and new ones replace them because, before a cell dies, it divides. The moment a cell is created, its death (*apoptosis*) is already genetically determined. When it divides, it passes on genetic information to the new cell, such as its appearance, its task, its frequency of division, and its life span. A cell's life cycle extends from its creation to its division and finally to its death.

If something goes wrong in this very complicated process, a degenerate cell arises. This cell may just die, or it may divide repeatedly, producing more degenerate cells. You then have a tumor, which is really just a clump of "wrong" cells. The creation of a tumor can be caused by many outer factors. Alcohol, nicotine, vitamin deficiency, harmful substances in food, environmental poisons, radiation, and viruses can eventually affect normal cell division in a harmful way. So can inner factors such as stress or emotional strain. And finally, some forms of cancer arise through hereditary predisposition.

If you consider that millions of cells tread their daily predetermined path of growth, division, and death, it is obvious that "accidents" may occur in parts of the body, and that tumor cells may arise. If everything goes normally, our immune system is designed to handle these. For example, white blood cells (leukocytes) recognize cell debris (such as tumor cells) and destroy them by literally eating them up. However, the process doesn't function well if there are too many degenerate cells for the leukocytes to destroy successfully, or because the immune system is too weak.

Tumor Cells

A tumor can be benign or malignant; often only so diagnosed after it has been surgically removed and investigated. About eighty percent of all breast tumors are benign. It is a characteristic of tumors that their cells keep dividing and increasing. Tumors can become invasive, growing into surrounding tissues or organs (infiltration), hindering and eventually killing them, because the tumor needs ever more room to grow.

For many oncologists, malignant tumors—the most important of which are called carcinomas, according to their origin—become the focus of cancer treatment. They must be removed. After that, if patients show no further signs of the cancer, they are considered healed—that is, if the tumor does not reappear within five years. However, there may be more than one tumor during the course of a disease. Remember, a tumor can arise from a single degenerate cell. If a cell separates from the original primary tumor, it can get swept elsewhere via the circulatory or lymph system. On its journey it is either destroyed by a leukocyte or it settles in an organ or lymph node and forms a daughter tumor (*metastasis*).

Our body consists of thousands of different cells, so you can imagine how many kinds of carcinoma might arise. Some of these grow very slowly and don't disperse (they don't metastasize). Some grow rapidly but are not widely dispersed. Others don't form solid tumors; instead they become cancer of the blood (leukemia) or lymph glands (lymphomas, Hodgkin's disease).

To form an idea of the frequency of various carcinomas, please look at the following chart. It lists the six most common forms of cancer (not the number of deaths). In that connection the following should be mentioned:

- In the last twenty years the number of colorectal cancer cases has increased more rapidly than any other cancer.
- Even men can get breast cancer, although rarely.
- The carcinomas listed appear much more often in people over sixty years of age, but there are a few rare kinds that appear only or mainly in children.
- Each sex has its own carcinomas (uterine cancer in women, prostate cancer in men) but most cancers make no distinction between men and women.

Cancer: More than a Tumor: Effects on General Health

At first a tumor can cause a lot of discomfort, or none at all. A rapidly growing tumor can cause increasing pain to its host, leading to death in a few short weeks. A slow-growing breast carcinoma may remain undiscovered for ten years or more and still be painless after it is found. The severity of pain depends both on the kind of tumor the patient develops and the stage of the disease.

Aside from the direct effects, cancer has other, far-reaching implications. It impacts not just the diseased organ but the whole person. Cancer patients often feel physically weak and tired. Colds and other infections frequently plague them and aren't overcome as quickly as before. This is because the immune system is weakened and the leukocytes cannot function properly.

What we call our general health has physical, psychic, spiritual, and social aspects. All of them are closely interrelated. Patients often say that "their world collapsed" when the doctor told them they had cancer. At first, they fall into a black hole: *How far has the cancer progressed? Are there any metastases? What are my chances of being cured?* Questions like these preoccupy

---

Number of New Malignancies per Year (US 1999)[1]

Four million patients are currently treated for cancer each year, while 1.22 million are newly diagnosed.

Types of Cancer

Prostate	179,300
Breast	176,300
Lung	171,600
Colorectal	129,400
Bladder	54,200
Stomach	21,900

and plague the individual during the first days after the initial diagnosis.

Doctors cannot always be certain about the prospects for successful treatment; they can often only offer estimates based on experience and current statistics.

Strains on the patient's general condition are compounded during the course of the disease. Even the treatments discussed later in this chapter can tax a person to the physical limits, which in turn will affect the soul. Cancer patients often suffer from wide mood swings, ranging from euphoria (I'll make it!) to hopelessness (I have only two more weeks to live). If you con-

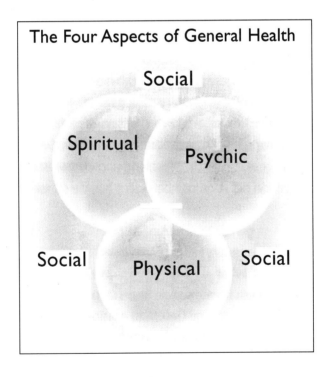

The Four Aspects of General Health

Social

Spiritual

Psychic

Social

Physical

Social

sider how strongly moods affect our general physical health, you can see that cancer is far more than just a tumor.

Indeed, you may well be familiar with this situation: You suddenly hear that a friend or colleague has been diagnosed with cancer. You want to visit and offer help, but you are uncertain. Should you broach the subject or wait until it is mentioned? Should you talk about death and pain or should you avoid the topic altogether, and speak in a lighter vein? Everyone experiences this uncertainty in dealing with the seriously ill. Even doctors don't always find the right approach.

Of course the patient immediately notices that the relationship with family, friends, and colleagues changes, and perhaps becomes inhibited. Acquaintances, because of their own uncertainties, sometimes may even avoid the patient. Feelings of loneliness and segregation set in, which can be intensified by the treatment itself. A patient who experiences hair or weight loss during chemotherapy or radiation sometimes suffers more from stares on the street than from the severe physical effects of the treatment. Both the physical and psychological strains of having this illness can weaken a person's constitution, even when the carcinoma itself isn't directly responsible.

We all know that we cope better with hardships of all kinds when we are mentally stable. Cancer can unhinge even the most balanced person, because the disease usually brings about such a radical change in personal and professional life. Tens of thousands of people become unfit for work yearly. This impacts the economy as well as the patient, which makes us aware of the larger social dimension of the illness.

Cancer patients tend to withdraw from other people at first. And because we live in a society of healthy people in which there is little room for our sick, it becomes difficult for the latter to cultivate their usual social connections and to retain the very important feeling of being of value to family, friends, and colleagues. If this feeling is suddenly undermined because of cancer, life becomes empty, and the psychological foundation necessary for a return to good health is lacking.

Intellectual or spiritual work adds dimension and importance to people's lives. A patient lying in hospital with a broken leg can use the time to catch up on reading, writing, or contemplation. In these situations, the general intellectual or spiritual condition is not adversely affected. A cancer patient, however, frequently complains of feeling spiritually washed out and no longer capable of completing tasks, or of absorbing things. Cancer's invasiveness goes beyond general health to affect intellectual and spiritual health.

While eliminating the growth of the tumor is of primary importance, strengthening all aspects of the patient's general state of health is often the decisive factor in successful cancer treatment. Patients' prospects are better if they are in good physical condition, psychologically balanced, and socially and spiritually active. Achieving and maintaining overall good health is the basis of integrative cancer treatment as described in this book.

Tumor Therapy

The first question a patient asks is: "Is it benign or malignant?" Many ways lead to the initial discovery of a tumor. Examples are:

- A change in the size or color of a birth mark or the size of a nodule in the breast;
- Complaints about digestive disturbances or problems with urination;
- A breast or prostate checkup revealing a suspicious growth.

Once a tumor is discovered, careful, well-considered action is required. Depending on the kind and location of the tumor, the doctor will conduct tests to determine whether the cancer is malignant or benign, and to classify it. Various methods of investigation are available.

A *blood sample* can often reveal a great deal. Laboratory doctors can determine the tumor's immune status by counting the number and kind of defensive cells contained in the blood. One way our immune system reacts to particular tumors is to form quantities of special defensive cells. In addition, most tumors betray themselves through so-called *markers*. These are substances such as hormones, proteins, or various cells. These are either formed by the tumor, or the tumor induces the body to build them. If the laboratory finds a high PSA (prostate specific antigen) value in a blood sample, it is a marker—a sign—that indicates the presence of a benign or malignant disease of the prostate.

Seven Signs of Possible Cancer

1. Any wound or ulcer that doesn't heal.
2. Nodules and thickenings in or under the skin, especially in the mammary gland area, and large swellings in lymph nodes.
3. Any change in a mole or birthmark
4. Ongoing stomach problems, difficulty swallowing, or intestinal irregularities.
5. Long term coughing or hoarseness
6. Bloody feces, urine, sputum, or other unusual excretions from the body orifices.
7. Irregular menses and bleeding after menopause.

Finding and Assessing a Tumor

In addition to markers, there are a number of visual aids with which to diagnose the presence of a tumor. Depending on location and complexity, a physician may use

- X-ray (sometimes with a dye that helps to provide a better look at particular parts of the body);
- Sonogram, which does not stress the body as much as X-rays;
- Computer tomography (CT) or magnetic resonance tomography (MRT), a relatively expensive method of diagnosis that provides three-dimensional pictures of the tumor as well as a speedy and accurate assessment of it; and

- Scintigraphy, in which the patient gets an injection of a radionuclide. The mild radiation is not dangerous, and the scintiscans can provide a very accurate picture of possible tumor foci through the distribution of radiating substance in blood vessels, tissues and organs.

Finally, a doctor may remove some of the irregular tissue (*biopsy*) to examine it histologically. *Histology* is the study of tissues. A microbiologist examines tissues in order to determine whether cells are benign or malignant, and to which kind of tumor they belong. If a biopsy is not possible, then the whole tumor must be surgically removed, and later subjected to a histopathological investigation.

The doctor tries to determine the level of malignancy of a tumor and its classification as soon as possible, although sometimes classification is only possible after treatment has begun, following the removal of the tumor. The classification summarizes the most important characteristics of the illness.

TNM Staging

"TNM staging," used internationally, is the most common classification system. This system permits doctors to classify essential tumor data with a short set of letters and numbers. T stands for tumor, N for node and M for metastases. A number follows each letter. TNM staging is slightly different for each kind of cancer. The table on the next page shows the classification for common breast cancer.

A doctor who reads "breast carcinoma T1N1Mo" knows that this tumor is up to two centimeters large, has one or more swollen lymph nodes, possibly affected, and no sign of metasta-

---

Histological Grading of Tumor Cells

G1   very well differentiated

G2   fairly well differentiated

G3   poorly differentiated

Gx degree of differentiation not determined

A tumor's degree of malignancy is determined by comparing the similarity of its cells to the surrounding healthy tissue. The greater the similarity, the better the differentiation and the less ·malignant the tumor.

---

sis. On the basis of this classification, a prognosis can be made. *A prognosis is a prediction about the course of the disease based on general statistics and worldwide experience with cancer.*

A patient may hear that "the prognosis is good" or "it's unfavorable." The doctor may give the patient a certain number of years to live, or relay other expectations. *These are statistical probabilities of healing, survival rates, and times for all types of cancer.*

A physician will immediately share a favorable statistical prognosis with the patient. But if the prognosis is not so favorable a doctor often keeps it to himself, responding only to urgent questioning. And he's right in doing so: *statistics are only probabilities, not facts or guarantees.* A patient with a particular type of cancer that has a ninety-nine percent death rate, statistically speaking, may belong to the one percent group that fully recovers.

TNM Classification for Breast Cancer

T Primary Tumor

Tis   Pre-invasive Carcinoma

T0   No basis for primary tumor

T1   Tumor diameter $\leq$ 2 cm

T2   Tumor > 2 cm < 5 cm

T3   Tumor $\geq$ 5cm

T4   Tumor of any size

N regional homolateral lymph nodes

N0   No palpable axillary lymph nodes

N1   Palpable, moveable axillary lymph nodes

N2   Lymph nodes attached to each other or to something else

N3   Supra- or infraclavicular nodes or arm edemas

M Metastasis

M0   No sign of metastases

M1   Existing metastases

Medical terms:

- Carcinoma in situ = pre-invasive
- Regional ipsiolateral = lymph node near the tumor on one side of the body
- Axillary = located in the arm pit
- Supra/infra clavicular = located above/under the collarbone

Because cancer is such a prevalent disease, stories of "medical miracles" often arise: a tumor suddenly stops growing and the patient dies of old age years later, with that tumor still in place but unchanged. Another patient experiences spontaneous remission for no apparent reason—the tumor shrinks, with or without treatment, disappears and never again causes problems. As you read on you will find many factors that affect healing, some of which were just mentioned. In any case, statistical prognosis makes a general statement about the totality of cancer patients and has no significance in the individual case.

Cancer Treatments

The Three Pillars of Conventional Cancer Therapy

Surgery, radiation, and chemotherapy make up the three classic pillars of conventional cancer treatment. The destruction of the tumor is their first and most important goal. Decades of use worldwide have yielded abundant experience, especially with the various components of chemotherapy, which undergo so-called clinical trials on an ongoing basis. These trials employ the *prospective, randomized, double blind studies* favored by orthodox medical science. A new medicine must be tested in such trials to be approved for distribution to, and acceptance by, physicians.

"Randomized" means that a large group of patients are randomly divided into two or more groups for a prospective study. This is meant to guarantee that each group has the same values or characteristics. During the trial one group receives the medication being tested, and the other group, or groups, receives an inert substance (*placebo*). "Double blind" means that neither the patients nor their own physician, nor the people conducting the study, know who has received the placebo and who the real medicine until after the trial is complete. This is to prevent bias, especially on the part of the patient.

Interestingly a *placebo effect* is fairly frequent. This means that patients taking the placebo experience symptoms and side effects as though they had been getting the real medication. This phenomenon can arise from many factors not related to the placebo alone. These factors might be other therapeutic measures conducted during the trial, or they may be psychosomatic and psychotherapeutic. The fact that placebo effects do arise at all in these clinical trials, and that they are difficult to explain, strongly indicates possible interactions between body and soul that are inaccessible to conventional scientific knowledge.

In cancer therapy such randomized, double-blind studies present a problem. Testing a treatment of which one expects good results means having to deny half of the patients this possibly life-saving intervention. There are many physicians, among them some anthroposophical doctors, who do not take part in such studies. Besides, such clinical trials can furnish only physical measurements in a relatively small number of candidates; if and how treatment affects the soul is very hard to standardize by such measures.

Soul effects are largely considered to be subjective, and "subjective measurements" do not easily fit into a conventional, scientific view of the world. This is why they are rarely investigated in clinical trials. Recently, however, a number of investigations have attempted to measure the quality of life—also a subjective factor. The influence of mistletoe therapy upon the quality of life of cancer patients has been, and continues to be, investigated, with very encouraging results, although some conventionally oriented doctors doubt the scientific basis of such studies.

Conventional cancer therapy is mainly directed at destroying the tumor, which it attacks in the three ways mentioned, either singly, or in pairs, or bundled in various combinations over time.

Surgery

There are countless techniques for removing a tumor. Some tumors can be removed through minimally invasive laparoscopic surgery. Depending on the type and stage of the illness, more comprehensive surgery, perhaps even amputation, may be called for. In every case, the surgeon will remove some healthy surrounding tissue to make sure that not a single cancer cell has been left behind.

If lymph nodes are diseased, they are removed, including healthy lymph nodes near a tumor. Tumors can appear anywhere, including places that are hard for a surgeon to reach. This applies to certain brain tumors, where one of the other two methods already mentioned must be used. Depending on where the tumor is found, radiation or chemotherapy may be indicated to shrink its size before attempting surgery. Conversely, a tumor that at first cannot be completely removed may be surgically reduced in size to give radiation or chemotherapy a better chance of dissolving it.

Chemotherapy

The second pillar of conventional cancer therapy is chemotherapy, which uses various medications called *cytostatics*. "Cyt" means "cell," and cytostatics work on the status or condition of the cell. They are cytotoxic, poisoning and destroying body cells. As we have already discussed, tumor cells are nothing but mutated, previously normal cells that divide and multiply faster than the cells they originated from. Cytostatics only destroy cells in the process of division. Just because cancer cells grow and divide more rapidly than normal cells, however, does not mean that cytostatic treatment destroys only cancerous tissue. Therefore, the physician chooses carefully calculated combinations of cytostatic substances that affect different stages of cell development, in an attempt to target the tumor cells while sparing the healthy cells as much as possible.

In certain cancers, such as prostate and especially those that do not form solid tumors such as leukemia or Hodgkin's, chemotherapy can be very effective, although the patient may suffer considerably from side effects during treatment. However, the prognosis is very good for these forms of cancer and justifies such radical therapy. In the end, the patient must participate in the choice of treatment he or she will be receiving, because ultimately they will be helping to *support* the treatment and not just enduring it.

Side effects impact especially the blood-forming system, which has to be monitored continuously during chemotherapy, and which is often on the verge of collapse. A patient's mucous membranes also suffer, and severe gastrointestinal disorders can result from chemotherapy. Because it regenerates itself so frequently, the skin is also affected. Chemotherapy patients often lose their hair (also called "skin appendages"). Because of these various physical side effects, patients may suffer from severe depression and other adverse psychological trauma.

> *Sadly, in the past, such interventions have not resulted in conclusive success. In some cases, good psychosocial care and widely based support treatments are more important than the medical therapy directed at the tumor.*[2]

Besides their use in cancer therapy, cytostatics are used in organ replacement therapy, because they suppress the body's immune system. With them, it is possible to prevent the body from recognizing the new organ as a foreign element and rejecting it. Any patient on chemotherapy has a weakened immune system, leading to life-threatening complications. Infections are the greatest danger; in some circumstances even a cold can be fatal.

While chemotherapy has a firm place in cancer treatment, and its responsible use is justified, some well respected physicians object to its excessive use:

> *After several decades of intensive clinical investigation of cytostatic substances there is still no evidence that chemotherapy gives patients with advanced stages of cancer a longer life expectancy.*[3]

Radiation Therapy

Radiation is the third strategy used by conventional medicine to destroy tumors. There are many reasons for using radiation therapy, such as after an operation to eliminate remaining cancer cells, or if a physician can't reach the tumor with a scalpel. Radiation is particularly suited for malignant, rapidly forming tumors because they are more sensitive to radiation than other bodily tissues and can sometimes best be destroyed with localized rays.

X-rays, gamma rays, and electron radiation are some of the many therapeutic radiation methods used today. But because all forms of radiation tend to destroy the body tissue they pass through, radiologists and nucleologists work out a radiation plan that is as exact as possible for each case. This helps ensure that the tumor is completely destroyed while the least possible damage is done to healthy tissue.

The skin reacts to radiation by displaying sunburn-like symptoms, including irritation, reddening, browning, and loss of hair at the radiated spots. The patient often feels generally unwell following treatment. Depending upon the treated organ or area, side effects can range from urination problems or intestinal inflammations: the side effects are not always temporary and, in rare cases, produce scars on affected organs. This can lead to irregularities in evacuation of the bladder and intestines.

Interactive Therapies

Treating the Tumor from Many Sides
The three classic pillars of cancer treatment are often used together or in pairs. Radiation or chemotherapy used in conjunction with surgery is called accessory (adjunct) treatment. It is meant to ensure that the tumor and possible metastases are completely destroyed.

Beyond these, there are many other adjuncts to treating cancer. Some are commonly used and generally accepted, while others are looked upon with doubt in conventional medical circles. Here are some examples.

Hormone Therapy
Today it is common knowledge that the growth of certain carcinomas is hormone dependent. The hormone estrogen has a growth regulatory effect on tumors in the female breast. The hormone hydroxy-progesterone influences endometrial cancer. Depending on the particular case, hormone or anti-hormone preparations can change the hormone balance of a patient to such an extent that metastases can be prevented, or the severity of the disease reduced (known as remission).

Biological Immune Therapy
As discussed earlier, leukocytes or natural killer cells in our immune system recognize tumor cells and destroy them. Biological immune therapies are meant to stimulate this function, or to harmonize the disrupted system. Today we know that a direct relationship exists between our central nervous

system, the immune system, and the soul. An immune therapy that considers these aspects can build resistance to the cancer, and strengthen and support a patient's energy and even the will to live. However, one should not rely solely on immune therapy for tumor destruction.

Therapy with Isolated Lectins

Medications have been on the market for some time now that are said to have a standardized content of mistletoe lectin 1 (ML1). It is assumed that ML1 and other ingredients of mistletoe have an inhibiting effect on tumor growth. The manufacturers of such lectin preparations say that ML1 is their only medically active ingredient. But, in fact, these medications are aqueous extracts of the whole mistletoe plant, and the ML1 activity is derived from a standardization of the total content of ML1, ML2, and ML3. These preparations may contain a certain quantity of ML1, but they also contain undetermined quantities of other substances. Lectin preparations may be quite suitable for adjunct tumor therapy, although theoretically not using the full therapeutic potential of all the substances in a mistletoe extract.

Homeopathic Medication

Very diluted (attenuated) homeopathic remedies are used to activate the body's own healing forces. Homeopathic medications can be drawn upon to treat many of the complaints that accompany cancer. A good homeopath would never claim that his or her treatment destroys tumors, for the treatment can only help to support the body's own functions. Homeopathy cannot treat tumors directly.

Mistletoe Therapy

An extract from the whole mistletoe plant contains various lectins (the main ones being ML1-3), numerous viscotoxins, and more. *In vitro* test tube experiments with these two groups of substances indicate that they have an inhibiting or lethal effect on cancer cells.

Mistletoe therapy has been used in Germany and Switzerland in the treatment of cancer for over eighty years. To date, about 30,000 patients have been treated with mistletoe at the Lukas Clinic in Arlesheim, Switzerland. About half of the physicians practicing in Germany now use mistletoe as adjunct therapy, and their numbers continue to increase. Many studies have tracked the good results experienced by patients (in vivo)that confirm the anti-tumor effects found in test tubes.

The most common form of mistletoe therapy is subcutaneous injection. It is relatively simple and can usually be done by the patient at home after the physician demonstrates the proper procedure. The mistletoe preparation is generally injected twice or three times a week with a very thin needle into the area prescribed by the physician. It is a procedure similar to the injection of insulin for diabetes. Mistletoe preparations can be given intravenously, but this is usually done in clinics or private practices that specialize in cancer or in hospitals with inpatient services.

Shortly after an injection, the patient usually experiences a local reaction, especially at the beginning of therapy. The skin

Substances Contained in Whole Mistletoe Extract and Their Effects on Tumor Cells

Mistletoe lectins and other glycoproteins	Cytotoxicity through inhibition of protein synthesis
Viscotoxins and other polypeptides	Cytotoxicity by dissolving cell membranes
Peptides	Cytotoxicity (tumor inhibition in the laboratory)
Polysaccharides	Inhibition of the cytotoxicity of mistletoe lectins
Oligosaccharides	Tumor inhibition in the laboratory

Definitions: ribosomal protein synthesis=the process by which a cell produces protein to form new cells/ induction of apoptosis=the induction of cell death.

at the puncture site gets red, warm, slightly swollen, and itchy for a short time. Local reactions do not appear in all patients after injections. The doctor will monitor the reaction to the first few injections and modify treatment if necessary; these reactions, however, are not dangerous.

That the organism responds positively to mistletoe therapy with a local reaction is desirable, as will be explained further in the following chapter. Besides its effect on the actual tumor, mistletoe has other positive aspects, from which an integrative approach to cancer treatment can benefit.

Anthroposophically Extended Medicine

The concepts of integrative cancer treatment, mistletoe therapy, and anthroposophically extended medicine are closely connected. Here is a brief explanation of anthroposophically extended medicines.

Rudolf Steiner (Austrian philosopher and scientist, 1861–1925) founded the Anthroposophical Society (Greek: human [*anthropos*] and wisdom [*sophia*]) in Germany in the early 1900s based on an epistemology and a spiritual scientific world view with the human being at its center. This world view has been widely influential since then, giving rise to Waldorf schools and kindergartens, and to various forms of therapeutic education. Biodynamic agriculture, which grows crops according to laws of nature and the cosmos in order to nourish the "whole" human being, has its origins in anthroposophy as well.

Steiner also gave medical indications to physicians. These indications were subsequently developed further. Today, anthroposophically extended medicine has a recognized place in the public health systems of Europe with a dozen clinics as well as several hundred doctors in private practice using these methods. A large teaching hospital at the University of Witten-Herdecke in Germany was founded through the initiative of anthroposophical doctors. It is also a medical school. So was the Lukas Clinic in Switzerland. Anthroposophically extended medicine is established worldwide from New Zealand to Brazil and Great Britain to the United States.

Collaboration in Cancer Treatment

Anthroposophically extended medicine does not promote rules that dictate a course of action to an anthroposophical physician. Therefore, the description of anthroposophically extended medicine cannot be expected to fit every physician.

First and foremost, the anthroposophical physician is a fully trained and licensed medical doctor who, like every other medical doctor, must be fully conversant with conventional medical practice. However, conventional medicine deals mainly with the physical body. This is just the starting point in anthroposophically extended medicine which understands the human being as a unity of body, soul, and spirit, including life phenomena, and consciousness with all degrees of feeling and self-awareness. These levels of existence are inseparably connected to each other. For the anthroposophical physician, illness never affects just the physical body—it affects the patient as a whole. The goal of anthroposophical medicine is to restore the harmony between levels of existence previously disrupted by illness, and to help the patient find a new balance in his or her environment.

Anthroposophical therapies such as therapeutic eurythmy treat not just the disease but the whole human being. An anthroposophical physician is not required to be a naturopath, although treatment with natural medicines and methods has its firm place in anthroposophically extended medicine, as does homeopathy. An anthroposophical physician may treat a broken toe just like any other doctor, but the more complicated the pathological process is, the more the doctor will take into account the patient's soul and consciousness in the choice of therapies.

If you are familiar with the ideas in holistic medicine you will know that many of them agree with the content of anthroposophically extended medicine. It can very well happen that a holistic doctor who has nothing to do with anthroposophical medicine may prescribe treatments similar to those an anthroposophical physician would choose.

It is vital to understand that anthroposophically extended medicine is not an alternative to conventional medicine, but rather a logical extension of it. It does not claim to always have the best or only path to healing. Anthroposophical medicine does, however, have the most experience with the use of mistletoe in cancer treatment, which is the theme of this book, although any physician can carry out skillful mistletoe therapy.

Mistletoe Therapy

An Achievement of the Anthroposophical Approach to Health and Illness

Over the last eighty-five years mistletoe has become the focus of attention in a new way. Once, Celtic Druids revered it as a general panacea for all ills. In the Middle Ages it was used for liver ailments and later on to lower blood pressure. Interest revived at the beginning of the 20th century. In 1907, the Munich-based botanist Karl von Tubeuf began to collect everything there was to know about mistletoe from mythology, cultural history, and natural science, and he published this as *Monographic der Mistel (Monograph on Mistletoe)* in 1923. In the fall of 1904, Rudolf Steiner began to speak about mistletoe within the framework of his spiritual scientific research activities.

The myths that surround mistletoe can be explained partly from its botanical qualities. Indeed, mistletoe is a unique plant. Although there are several varieties, only the mistletoe with white berries, *viscum album*, is used in cancer therapy. There are three subspecies of *viscum album* in central Europe: deciduous tree mistletoe, pine mistletoe, and spruce or fir mistletoe.

A unique trait of mistletoe is that it lives on host trees as a parasitic plant. Various kinds of birds eat its white berries, which contain one seed each. The birds either excrete the seed again and it sticks to a tree branch with their droppings, or they eat only the berry's flesh, leaving the uneaten seed sticking to a branch or tree trunk. The seedling then develops a sinker that penetrates the bark and wood of the host tree, through which the newly budding plant is able to get water and nourishment. The mistletoe bush has a distinct spherical shape and grows very slowly, only beginning to flower after five to seven years. When the plant is ten to fifteen years old, it is harvested and made into a medicine.

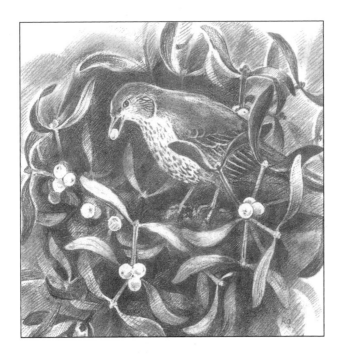

A New Task for an Ancient Plant

The Greeks called mistletoe "ixos" or "ixia." Iscador, also known as Iscar, are brand names for mistletoe tincture, and take their names from the Greek. Since 1935, the Society of Cancer Research in Arlesheim, Switzerland, has been concentrating all its efforts on the manufacture, research, and development of Iscador. The Lukas Clinic, founded in 1935 and an offshoot of the Society of Cancer Research, specializes in treating cancer patients with Iscador as well as with corresponding alternative therapies, many of which are discussed in this book.

As early as 1917, Rudolf Steiner suggested using injections of mistletoe extract for the treatment of cancer. His recommendation was taken up and put to clinical use by Ita Wegman, a

Dutch physician. Dr. Wegman, who founded a clinic in Arlesheim, developed Iscador, together with a growing group of clinical practitioners. Iscar the homeopathic version of Iscador, is available in the U.S. from Weleda, Inc., a Swiss-based homeopathic pharmaceutical company. Iscador is the most prescribed mistletoe preparation used today.

Any anthroposophical mistletoe preparation is by no means simply a pressed juice. As previously mentioned, the sap contains lectins, peptides, viscotoxins and other proteins, as well as polysaccharides. More research work on these ingredients is continually being done, but it is known that viscotoxins are cytolytic, that is they quickly dissolve the membrane of tumor cells. Mistletoe lectins act more slowly and cytostatically; that is, they inhibit the growth of tumor cells.

Mistletoe contains the greatest amount of viscotoxins in summer and the greatest amount of lectins in winter. Harvesting mistletoe both in spring and autumn provides sap from the same plant but with an emphasis on two different ingredients. The harvested mistletoe is carefully worked into a tincture by a special method, and then summer and winter saps are mixed together in a copper-lined centrifuge. The preparation that arises in this way contains some viscotoxins and some lectins, both of which have antitumoral effects, and also contains plenty of all the rest of mistletoe's ingredients. Much is still unknown about the latters' effects, but it seems that the effect of lectins and viscotoxins upon cancer is enhanced by these trace ingredients. "The whole is more than the sum of its parts," certainly applies to mistletoe therapy. This element of the intangible may be one of the reasons that most doctors trust this kind of mistletoe preparation more than preparations that contain simply isolated lectins.

Experiencing Life: Integrative Cancer Treatment

Conventional cancer treatment targets the tumor, which is diagnosed as precisely as possible and destroyed as quickly and radically as possible. Then the side effects of the tumor-destroying therapies are treated as effectively as possible. Successful treatment is followed by an after-care phase that is diagnostically oriented: by way of regular checkups, the doctor looks for signs of a relapse. This is the classic procedure if the destruction of the primary tumor and of all metastases present was successful.

Integrative cancer therapy goes beyond the destruction of a tumor. The patient's quality of life and other factors besides the tumor are also of considerable importance. Quality of life is composed of countless elements that are of varying importance to different people. Health is a very important factor for everyone; and it is endangered for a cancer patient. In integrative therapy the task is to find out *what other factors* are important to each individual patient and to strengthen and support these as much as possible. A patient's general feeling of well being consists of many dimensions. If it is good—aside from the cancer—a patient will be able to deal with the side effects of the tumor-destroying treatment better, recovery from the treatment will be easier and faster, and the chances of a relapse will be less.

Disease and Quality of Life

Various complementary, adjunct, and palliative measures can be taken to improve the patient's general condition and thereby the quality of life. Some of these have already been presented here in connection with tumor destruction. Mistletoe therapy has a very positive effect on the quality of life. You will learn more about this on the following pages.

Unfortunately, a complete and successful destruction of a tumor is often not possible. The disease may be at a stage where removing the tumor and/or all metastases is no longer possible, or the primary tumor quickly recurs in the patient.

Then there is the question everyone associated with cancer asks: How long will I live and how will the remaining time be? You already know that conventional medicine can only answer these questions statistically, but this does not necessarily have binding relevance in the individual case. The second part of the question concerns quality of life, which can be improved considerably through the use of mistletoe in an integrative therapy. Indeed, it is often necessary to weigh the importance of the different quality of life factors for each individual patient to get the best possible results of an "individualized" therapy.

For example, palliative pain therapy can increase or restore the quality of life to a patient experiencing a great deal of pain from conventional cancer therapy, because the absence of pain is an important quality of life factor. But such a palliative therapy may have to include high doses of strong analgesics, so that the patient has trouble concentrating and feels "numb" and as if "packed in cotton." He or she can't read with much concentration anymore or participate animatedly in conversations with friends or relatives. In this case the quality of life "freedom from pain" takes precedence over other qualities of life such as "intellectual capability" and "social competence."

Quality of Life

In Germany, research has shown that people look for improved quality of life. The following eighteen factors were considered most important although varying from one individual to the next:[4]

Sphere of activity: Do I have better mobility, can I travel more easily, is there enough infrastructure for me?

Employment: Are things going better for me in my economic situation, am I recognized for a particular activity (given respect)?

Food: Is my food wholesome and tasty? Does it improve my intellectual output and my mood?

Feeling Life: Am I full of optimism, hope, joy in life, comfort, security, sympathy, and love?

Intellectual Capacity: Is my concentration and learning ability growing?

Social Life: Are my relations with family, partner, friends and trusted people improving?

Feeling of Well Being: Am I free of pain, symptoms and problems?

Freedom from Conflicts: Are my conflicts decreasing?

Body Control: Are my mobility and elasticity improved?

Communication: Do I have more possibilities of exchanging ideas and of gaining recognition?

Cultural Knowledge: Do I have better possibilities of cultural experiences, or am I already surrounded by culture? Is my perception of beauty and aesthetics improving?

Social Responsibility: for children, family, partner, neighbors, friends, trusted people, oppressed and needy people, and all humankind—is it improving?

Sleep, Rest: Is there enough energy, and do I have an unrestricted source of strength?

Vacation, Relaxation: Are my free time and hobbies being promoted?

Awareness of the Environment: Is ecology improving?

Living Quarters: Are my subjective living conditions improving?

Sexuality: Is my sex life improving?

Dying "Well": Am I finding calm inner peace, physical relaxation and spiritual acceptance?

In another example, a patient has cancer in an advanced stage and only expects to live another six months. The doctors think that chemotherapy would add another year to that. But chemotherapy would keep him or her from fulfilling an ardent wish to take one more trip to Australia. In such a case a choice has to be made between a lengthening of life "at any price" and the fulfillment of a "lifelong dream." A doctor can offer advice here, but it is the patient who has to make the final decision.

Integrative cancer therapy that uses mistletoe preparations in cases where the cancer no longer seems curable can help ease patients' remaining time, so they live it and don't just have to endure it. However, one must not deny that there are forms of cancer and courses of the disease in which medical skill can no longer help. In such cases the treatment must concentrate on relieving the patients' discomfort and on supporting them in every respect in the last days of their life.

Mistletoe and the General Physical Condition
As described, in addition to its regulatory effect on the immune system (immunomodulatory effect), mistletoe therapy has a concrete effect on tumor cells. The local reaction patients experience after a mistletoe injection indicates that the body is reacting positively to the therapy. The mistletoe preparation actually stimulates the body's immune system.

As already mentioned, the immune system fights all "foreign" cells, pathogens, and tumor cells—if the immune system is intact. Fever is a sure sign that the immune system is "running at full speed." In this case, it should only be reduced if the temperature gets so high that it becomes life threatening. A patient's temperature increases slightly, sometimes even into the fever zone, after an injection of mistletoe and drops again in six hours or less. The weakness and headache and aching limbs that often accompany fever usually don't occur.

Changes in the immune system can be tracked through blood analysis; the number of neutrophile granulocytes (one of the many kinds of defensive cells in the immune system) increases considerably after the mistletoe injection and is still a little high the next day. Conversely, lymphocytes (another group of defensive cells that includes the natural killer cells that are especially desirable in cancer therapy) decrease in number, become normalized again, and then increase greatly after twenty-four hours. This immune modulating effect of mistletoe therapy is useful in cancer therapy in three ways:

1. The body's defense against circulating cancer cells is supported, which can prevent (further) metastases.

2. Surgery, radiation, and especially chemotherapy can greatly weaken the immune system. This weakening is partially eliminated through a simultaneous mistletoe therapy. Of course, an immune system that has been suppressed by "hard" chemotherapy cannot always be completely reharmonized again through mistletoe therapy.

3. After a successful tumor-destroying treatment, a bolstered immune system helps prevent relapses (recurrent prophylaxis) in the after-care phase. If the tumor was not completely healed or eradicated, the mistletoe therapy also provides better protection against infectious diseases in general.

An important general goal of anthroposophical therapy is the harmonizing—or reharmonizing—of a person's life processes, and experience has shown that mistletoe therapy can provide strong support here. Many cases document such harmonizing results: Mistletoe therapy can counteract the lack of appetite that is often connected with cancer, and enable patients to eat enough to get back to their normal weight. Mistletoe therapy can normalize disrupted sleep rhythms; sufficient, deep, refreshing sleep is very important for a cancer patient. Mistletoe

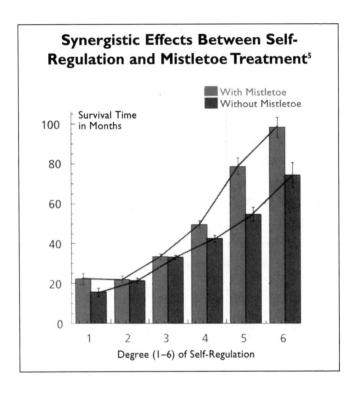

therapy can normalize disturbed blood-pressure regulation, stabilize blood pressure and improve both blood circulation and
its immune cells in the body.

Patients with cancer in advanced stages often say that they
experience less pain during mistletoe therapy. This may be
because of a stimulation of the body's endorphins. Endorphins
are substances formed by the body that kill pain—like mor-
phine—and make one feel "happy."

These physical effects of mistletoe therapy do not always
occur but are frequently observed and are reported in studies.
The full range of mistletoe therapy has still not been fully uti-

lized, but intensive work continues to be done. In future, you may expect much of mistletoe.

The Importance of Self-Regulation

The connection between the soul (psyche) and a person's physical condition is largely inexplicable, but everyone knows it exists. Psychic stress has been seen as a possible factor in triggering cancer. The pathological fear of getting cancer—carcinophobia—is a drastic example of the connection between body and soul. Even if the fear does not arise because someone's relatives or acquaintances have cancer, there is a high probability that a person with carcinophobia will indeed contract the disease.

Unfortunately, the converse is not true. People who have no fear of cancer develop it anyway. But the survival rate of cancer patients is distinctly lengthened if they are in good control of their soul (psychic self-regulation).

What is self-regulation? Self-regulation is the capacity to bring about one's own well being, inner equilibrium and a feeling of competency, and to cope with stressful situations. To put it very simply, having good self-regulation means being able to generate a "good feeling" in oneself and to create an inner harmony even when confronted by stress factors.

In a thirty-year study recently published, over 10,000 cancer patients with mostly advanced stages of cancer were investigated. Their self-regulation was tested and assessed with a comprehensive questionnaire (see graph on previous page). The result was clear: the better the patients' self-regulation abilities were, the longer they survived the disease, regardless of which therapy they had undergone. In a study investigating the effectiveness of mistletoe therapy on 1,000 patients, there was an increased average survival time from thirty-six to fifty-two months with mistletoe therapy. Another interesting result of this study was that the patients who underwent the mistletoe therapy had a higher degree of self-regulation than those who did not. Mistletoe therapy and good self-regulation complement each other.

Here again, statistics do not always apply to a single case. A patient with poor self-regulation abilities who does not undergo mistletoe therapy might nevertheless have a long survival rate, but these cases are rare.

One very interesting question that was not investigated in the study asks why mistletoe therapy patients develop better

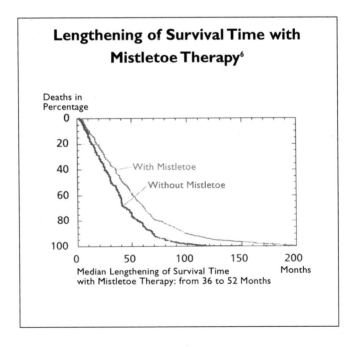

Lengthening of Survival Time with Mistletoe Therapy[6]

Deaths in Percentage

With Mistletoe

Without Mistletoe

Median Lengthening of Survival Time
with Mistletoe Therapy: from 36 to 52 Months

Months

self-regulation abilities than others. Researchers will surely pursue this question and perhaps be able to explain scientifically what still seems puzzling and mysterious today. In any case, studies have shown that the subjective quality of life of cancer patients is greater *during* mistletoe therapy than *before* therapy began. A new study of doctors using mistletoe will focus on this question. Perhaps additional indications as to the connections between self-regulation and mistletoe will emerge from it.

Other Complementary Cancer Treatments

The primary goal in conventional cancer treatment is to destroy any tumors that are found. If this is successful, steps must then be taken to guarantee both a speedy recovery and the best possible protection against relapses. If the cancer cannot be eliminated, integrative therapies can lengthen the patient's survival time, and help ensure that the patient can experience a high level of quality of life. The key phrase here is "quality of life."

The use of mistletoe *is* the basis of an integrative cancer therapy, but there is a lot more that can be done. The following are just a few examples of the kinds of therapeutic measures that can be used to supplement a combination of conventional cancer treatment and mistletoe therapy. For more information, please contact the phone numbers in the resource section, which is at the back of this guide.

Rhythmical Massage, developed by Ita Wegman, MD
The goal of rhythmical massage is to stimulate the immune system through positive skin stimulation. As a complementary

measure it is especially suitable for patients whose immune system has been weakened by chemotherapy or other strong treatments.

Therapeutic Eurythmy

In therapeutic eurythmy, words or tones are transposed into movements in space to attain a harmony with the organism's inner movements and to stimulate the organism's life forces. Therapeutic eurythmy has distinct meditative references, and can help one to renew one's inner self. It allows patients whose life has become disjointed because of the disease to become calm again, and helps activate the recovery process.

Artistic Therapies

Clay modeling, painting, music, and other artistic therapies are used in anthroposophical medicine to restimulate the patient's creativity. Patients who have already become resigned to the disease are encouraged to interact actively and creatively with their surroundings again, and to discover new energy needed to reshape life. Joy in artistic activity and in the results of one's own work can have positive effects on self-regulation.

Physical Therapy

Remedial gymnastics and mobility training can help bedridden patients quickly get back on their feet and deliberately get rid of physical deficiencies, such as weakness from lack of movement. When restriction of movement is a result of amputation or other radical surgery, general movement can be improved by the physiotherapies mentioned. Lymph drainage can eliminate congestion in the lymph system. The lymph system has to function perfectly if the immune system is to remain intact.

Sports

Movement is almost always healthy, regardless of the kind of cancer one has. It can strengthen the whole body as well as the immune system. In the preface to this chapter you read about a Tour de France winner who had been a cancer patient not too long before the race. Danish soccer forward Ebbe Sand had a similar fate: At twenty-six, he was operated on for testicular cancer, and yet twenty days later he was back on the field. These examples are motivational, and show what determination and strength of will can overcome. However, every cancer patient should consult a physician about the kind of sport he or she may play and the stresses involved.

Nutrition

Because of the severity of some of the conventional treatments, cancer patients are often underweight. To help counteract any nutrition deficiencies, patients should be sure to have a balanced diet. However, cancer in the liver or digestive organs and other factors can make it difficult to ensure this. It is advisable to discuss nutrition with the doctor.

Eating a lot of vitamins and minerals will support the immune system, but sufficient amounts of these elements are present in very nutritious food. The American Cancer Society has provided guidelines for a diet that may help reduce the risk of getting cancer. Every cancer patient should take them to heart: Don't get too fat or too thin; keep the fat portion of your food under thirty percent; make sure you eat a well-balanced diet that includes biodynamic or organic foods rich in vitamins, minerals, and trace elements; eat a lot of roughage; and avoid alcohol as much as possible.

Biofeedback and Self-training

These disciplines teach the techniques of relaxation. Relaxation is recommended for very restless and nervous patients, and is helpful to those patients who suffer from sleeping disorders and other forms of unrest.

The Simonton Method

Used when a patient is in a deeply relaxed state, this method involves the psychotherapeutic technique of "intrapersonal visualization" developed by Carl Simonton. For instance, an experienced therapist gets a deeply relaxed patient to visualize that he's sending out healthy cells that overcome the tumor and destroy every bit of it. A therapist certified in the Simonton Method must administer this therapy.

Yoga

Yoga has strong meditative qualities and can generate an "inner equilibrium" along the lines of a relaxation technique. Yoga increases the awareness of the body. Cancer patients who are plagued by stress can come to rest through yoga; they learn to "turn things off" and to find themselves.

Psychotherapy

Psychotherapy—alone or in a group—can help a patient develop positive strategies to cope with the fears and conflicts of the disease, and strengthen self-regulation abilities. Patients who discover or suspect deficiencies in self-regulation can make valuable contributions toward the standard treatment with a corresponding therapy.

Self-help Groups

In the United States, there is an almost blanketing network of self-help groups for cancer patients and even specific groups for those who suffer from different kinds of carcinoma. Patients whose disease has gotten them into new situations with which they can't cope, such as having to wear an artificial outlet for the intestines or bladder, can find others in their group with the same problems. By joining such a group, the patients realize they're not alone. Patients also benefit from valuable tips on how to deal with the illness, and may even be able to offer advice to a fellow group member, which helps raise self-esteem.

Social Activity

Going to a party or other social event can sometimes be of therapeutic value to a cancer patient. The social withdrawal that cancer patients sometimes choose has already been described here. But being human also includes the social aspects of life; conversation and interaction with others belong to life and are a big help in training or retaining the capacity for a healthy self-regulation.

These examples of complementary measures within the framework of an integrative cancer therapy cover only a fraction of therapies possible. Other measures not presented here might be suitable as well, depending on the patient's personality but also on the type and stage of the disease. Cancer is such a comprehensive theme that this guide can provide only a beginning impetus to becoming better informed. As mentioned in the preface, there are questions about cancer treatment that many doctors do not like to decide by themselves. To help the physician make the right decisions for a particular individual, the patient himself or herself needs to develop a comprehensive knowledge about the illness.

This section has listed fundamentals of integrative cancer treatment, based on anthroposophical mistletoe therapy as carried out by a physician. The next chapter examines commonly asked questions, and the following chapter will provide a list of resources.

Translated from "Mistel und Mehr"

1. American Cancer Society, www.cancer.org
2. Huhn, D, Herrmann, R [Hrsg.]: *Medical Therapy for Malignancies*. Foreword, Third Edition., G. Fischer, Stuttgart, Germany 1995
3. Abel, U, *Cytostatic Chemotherapy of Advanced Epithelial Tumors*. A Critical Case History, Foreword, Hippokrates, Stuttgart, Germany, 1990
4. Wilkes, M.W.: *The Economic Miracle. New Game Leadership. The Finding of New Markets and Market Regulations*, Frankfurt/Main, 1999
5. Grossarth-Maticek, R.: *A Prospective Study of Intervention*, Heidelberg,
6. Ibid.

Cancer—Disease of our Time

Rita Leroi, MD
and Walther Buehler, MD

TIME AND AGAIN DOCTORS ARE ASKED: "What really is the cause of cancer?" Obviously this question can't be answered in a single sentence. The increase in incidences of cancer indicates that the disease is related to our changed customs and living conditions—in the final analysis to our present image of the human being and the world. We, and with us our environment, have changed profoundly over the last hundred years. Rapid development has taken place, with which insight and a sense of responsibility have not always kept pace. This has contributed to a web of causes of why we are susceptible to cancer.

If we search for the actual cause of tumor formation only in the degenerate cell, or in the "accident" of hereditary or environmental factors, we are expressing a materialistically narrow view, detached from the soul-life of the human being. Even where demonstrable external factors, such as chemicals hostile to the organism, are identified, our constitution and individual susceptibility, or power of resistance, is always the deciding factor. Only by understanding the whole human being can we free ourselves of the fear that we are helplessly at the mercy of some accident in the cellular processes of our organism.

The human body is a well-formed, wisely constituted, organism whose building blocks are the cells. However, higher forces and principles of organization make the individual human form possible; they balance the relationship between shape and substance (cells). Today, we know a range of causes that disturb this balance and create the conditions for cancerous growth.

Disturbances of the Body

On the highest level, a disturbance can begin with the creative human spirit, if it is not given enough room to unfold in either education or profession. The spirit can become stunted and no longer master over its physical form. Disturbances can also occur in the life of the soul, in complexes, fears, and obsessions. These disturbances influence the harmonious function of our feeling life, the bodily basis of which is the rhythmic system of heart and lung. Finally, there can be disturbances in the body's metabolism, in the hormonal system, which can eventually lead to certain groups of cells breaking loose.

Preventive Help in Childhood

Preventive measures to ward off cancer can begin in pregnancy when the mother-to-be prepares herself physically and mentally with a rhythmic ordering of the day, sufficient sleep, a harmonious state of mind, avoidance of nicotine and alcohol, and healthy natural food.

Breast milk is the infant's best protection, not only because of the nutritive quality, but also for its vital formative forces. Breast milk strengthens the baby's basic constitution for the rest of its life. Giving the newborn a variety of substances foreign to mother's milk may lead to premature hardening or calcification, as do shots such as Vitamin D, which should not be given for mere reasons of prevention. Equally, excessive vaccinations in the early days should be avoided. Overcoming feverish childhood illnesses strengthens the immune system, and enables it, in later life, to resist attack.

Wholesome Education

It may seem strange at first that education is significant in preventing cancer. The key to understanding this idea, however, is a fundamental spiritual truth—that human thought forces are transformed growth forces. As the child develops, formative forces active in organic depths become free and are placed at the disposal of the ego as powers of memory and imagination. By stressing early reading, rote learning, and abstract thinking, we rob the very young child of just those forces, still needed for the body's formation, and prematurely put them in the service of the intellect. When this happens the child not only suffers from nervousness, loss of color and appetite, but the finer structures of the inner organism degenerate and threaten to harden and age before their time. Likewise, if creative imagination, artistic faculties, and inspired sharing of experiences are not sufficiently activated, there is a danger of damming up unused formative forces. These can later find expression in unhealthy behavior or unhealthy growth.

Today, an education that overemphasizes intellectual achievement and a lack of artistic expression are often the norm, and this education, unsuited to the developing child, can pave the way for tomorrow's ailments. Tragically, the earliest seeds of many pre-cancerous conditions often reach back into early childhood or schooling.

The middle school years should seek to *strengthen the individuality* of the child, at the same time awakening affectionate interest in the surrounding world. The *diet* of a school child is crucial and should be simple, but the food should be of biodynamic or organic quality. Young people should find *meaning in their work*, engaging themselves fully so their emerging personality permeates the organism that is their body in a healthy way, ordering and forming it.

* * *

Preventive Measures For Adults

Keeping a Rhythm

Tumors do not "breathe" normally. They demonstrate a "metabolism of suffocation." Conceived of this way, cancerous tumors lead us to look at the entire breathing process, a basic life rhythm united with the rhythm of the heart that carries the balance between organization and substance, between human form and cell. Every disturbance or weakening of this rhythm of life has a long-term damaging effect. In our present environment, far removed from the rhythms of nature, we are almost always exposed to such disturbances.

To help balance the unavoidable disruptions of everyday life, conscious care of the rhythmic system and penetrating the whole organism with breathing are important. Artistic activity, music, painting, eurythmy, and gardening, effectively nurture the rhythmic system, helping it remain pliant and lively.

Special care should be taken with the rhythm of waking and sleeping, which can be seen as the in- and out-breathing of our soul and spirit. Seven to eight hours sleep are sufficient for an adult, with one or two hours before midnight, when sleep depth is greatest. Meals should be regular, with a relaxed, cheerful mood prevailing. Bowels must be kept active with exercise, a good diet or, if necessary, with a mild vegetable laxative.

Warmth

More than with any other illness, people suffering from cancer see themselves as confronting an *opponent,* in the form of a growth, which to the patients' mind seems to lead them inexorably to the abyss of existence. Even experienced doctors keep wondering how such a separation between spirit-soul and the growth-ridden body can arise out of the original unity.

One answer is that what might be called the "warmth organism" falls apart. Through the medium of warmth, the ego permeates the body to its most distant fibers, giving it unity. For this reason, care and maintenance of a well-regulated warmth system is important. The gradual displacement of organs from this natural dynamic is one of the first factors predisposing the development of tumors. Rudolf Steiner suggested that a warm covering should be created around tumor activity to dissipate the illness and lead back to wholeness. This is perfectly logical. Steiner was the first to point to the polarity of inflammation and tumor growth. Living with a low temperature for years, the absence of inflammatory diseases, or the abrupt suppression of inflammatory diseases with fever-fighting drugs, are frequent signposts in the case history of a cancer-sufferer. One should not, therefore, avoid every little cold or minor fever with fever-lowering, germ-killing measures.

Many cancers arise in the abdomen. For the maintenance of a healthy flow of blood, this region must be not be allowed to get cold, in spite of the prevailing love of bare midriffs and legs, or thin nylons in cold weather, as well as synthetic clothing. These clothes contribute to the weakening of the unifying warmth organism, which in turn reflects back on the abdominal organs.

Strengthening the Ego
The ego is the spiritual essence that raises us above the animal kingdom to the rank of an individual with a complex healthy inner life. It is vital in the prevention of cancer. In modern life we are inwardly torn apart by a surfeit of external events—an over-abundance of sense impressions, freneticism, and a flood of unconnected bits of information from the media. All these cause constant stress and take far greater strength to meet than

the average person is capable of. As an antidote, we need to learn to acquaint ourselves with one small part of the world by experiencing it peacefully and deeply.

We must also practice growing old in the right way. Tissues harden physiologically with age but, as bodily capacities recede, the spiritual in theory is all the better able to unfold. Unfortunately, the opposite is often the case: the physical bodies of the elderly are artificially kept potent with hormones. Cancer, as a typical disease of old age, can arise precisely when aging tissue is artificially kept young, or when a cell imbalance arises through a chronic irritation in a particular area such as the alimentary tract. All interference in hormonal balance is harmful, and that includes the "Pill," which may encourage a disposition toward cancer when used over the long term. Combating hot flashes in menopause with hormones is to be avoided. On the other hand, everything possible should be done to keep what is spiritual alive, widening the horizons and unfolding the wisdom of old age.

Equally harmful is another kind of pill, the sedative, used to help people avoid every difficulty in life. Habitual use promotes a weakening of the will and also of the personality. Sleeping pills work in the same way. Both produce a slightly lowered consciousness and, even if not perceived, a weakening of initiative and tendency toward uniformity. Such a state is particularly susceptible to cancer.

Early Diagnosis

Regular medical examinations are strongly recommended for the recognition of pre-cancerous conditions. To this end, the development of special research methods arising out of anthroposophical medicine have been developed over many years, helping detect predisposition before the cancer develops to a physical stage. The copper chloride crystallization tests by *Pfeiffer* and the capillary-dynamic blood tests of *Kaelin* should be mentioned in this connection.

Treatment

A common reaction of patients in whom cancer has been diagnosed is: "I have always lived a healthy life. How could this happen to me?" Every disease is a part of our individual human destiny and belongs to us just as our arms and legs do. If we look back at the experiences of our lives up to the present, taking in all the good and all the bad, there is no part we would really want to leave out. Our personal biography is the garment of our earthly existence. The idea that our present life on earth is just one of many, a short step on the path of our individuality through earthly and spiritual stages, allows every life to be seen as a task, of which disease is a part, and one from which we can grow, regardless of the outcome. This is especially so with cancer. It constitutes a call to the sufferer: change thyself!

Surgery and radiation have made great strides in recent decades. Both methods, however, call for additional new directions in therapy since they only address the already degenerate cells. As early as 1920, Rudolf Steiner suggested a new therapy, based on his comprehensive insight into the nature of the human being and the natural world. With the introduction of mistletoe into cancer therapy, Steiner appealed to a new healing principle, that of addressing the forming forces of the organism (now called powers of resistance, or immune forces) which have the ability to control cell material gone wild.

In the meantime biochemical and biophysical research has shown that particularly strong tumor-inhibiting substances are contained in mistletoe extract. And so, in addition to the usual measures, we have today the possibility of extending and saving life with natural preparations made of mistletoe (*viscum album*). Even in situations where it is too late for surgery and where very little can be achieved with radiation, Iscador and the other mistletoe preparations may bring relief and added quality of life.

The Lukas Clinic in Arlesheim, Switzerland (one of a number of anthroposophical hospitals in Europe) specializes in the treatment and aftercare of people suffering from tumors, and uses Iscador and other adjunct therapies that address the whole human being. This rehabilitative treatment continues for years, even after the patient has left the clinic and returned to work.

Originally translated for LILIPOH from Sozial Hygiene, *Nos. 19 and 26, Helios Enterprises Ltd, Northbridge, Australia, with kind permission of the Verein für ein Anthroposophisches Heilwesen, Germany.*

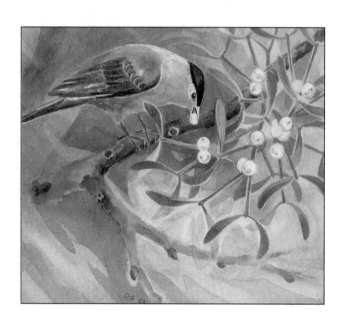

The Mysterious Shape of Mistletoe

Christine Murphy

ACCORDING TO THE DOCTRINE OF Signatures (Paracelsus), it is possible to see a plant's healing properties by the way it looks and behaves, its "signature," Mistletoe mimics cancer as a saprophyte, attaching itself to a host tree. Its lifestyle is irregular, too; fruiting in the middle of winter. Yet, it possesses a form which bespeaks lawfulness; as such is an image for overcoming the wild chaos of the disease.

Mistletoe is an alien, an outsider in the plant world and a visitor, as it were, from an earlier Earth development. It never touches the ground, growing on the branches of certain trees. It makes no effort to develop form and color in its floral organs, and its growth cycle is slow and the reverse of the normal plant cycle.

Higher plants take their first step into life on Earth by developing a root, which penetrates deep into the soil. Mistletoe also penetrates its "soil," the branch of the host tree, to begin with; but as soon as the bark has been passed and the delicate, living cambium is reached, the process no longer moves toward the center. From then on, the joining lets the wood of the host form a wall around it and mistletoe then grows out toward the periphery as the branch thickens.

Foliage development, normally rich and differentiated in "normal" plants, and rising toward the sun, is slow and simple in mistletoe. Each stem produces only one pair of leaves per year, and these look like undeveloped cotyledons (seed leaves). A mistletoe bush looks like a community of seedlings. Refusing to accept the developmental tendencies of the plant world in general, mistletoe always seeks to achieve its own special form— into a sphere. The two leaflets first lie close together, like hands folded in prayer. Then they gradually open, the angle between them growing until late autumn, when the two leaves are like a chalice. Next May, they are at right angles to the stem. Then they widen and stretch once more, the angle between leaf tips moving through the circle's arc with continuously extending radius. By the time the leaves, still green, drop off in August, the radius has extended full circle.

From the third year on, the stem of the young mistletoe plant begins to branch. The process is firmly guided to create a scaffolding in a sphere whose full form is achieved after seven years.

In March, when flowering is over, a third sphere begins to evolve. The undifferentiated female flower lengthens into a cylinder. The middle part gradually expands, with growth at the base, and tip held back, so that an egg-shaped form develops. The fruit gets rounder and rounder until, in December, the berry changes inwardly and begins to shine more and more brightly. Countless tiny lipid droplets in the mucilage reflect the light of the sun. Mistletoe refuses to unfold and differentiate as other plants do. In the mature, fruit-bearing mistletoe plant countless spherical elements interpenetrate, bearing infinite potential. It is perhaps this cosmic quality which made it sacred to the ancient druids.

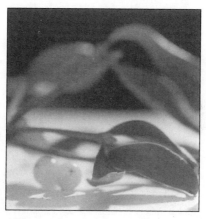

The mistletoe plant is harvested from a variety of host trees at midsummer time and during November/December.

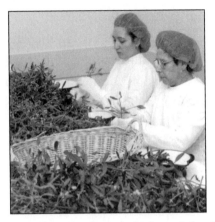

The plants are checked and cleaned by hand before selected parts undergo lactic acid fermentation.

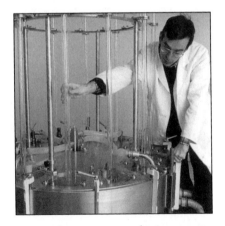

Twice a year, the summer and winter extracts are combined in a specially designed process for extraction of the natural medicine.

Treatment of Cancer with Iscador
A Physician's Answers to Frequently Asked Questions

Richard Wagner MD

ASED ON MANY DISCUSSIONS WITH MY patients, I believe it helpful to publish a short account of therapy with *Iscador*. During my eighteen years in practice, specializing in cancer treatment, I collected the most commonly asked questions. The following is an attempt to answer them in a concise way.

Despite research into the causes and treatment of cancer, pursued for many decades, contemporary oncology can only claim success in a few types of cancer. Among these are specific types of childhood leukemia, testicular carcinoma, specific sub-forms of mammary and lung cancer, lymphomas, Hodgkin's disease, and ovarian cancer. Yet, recent investigations show that, in the case of breast cancer, only few patients benefit from chemotherapy in a healing sense.

With many forms of cancer one has the impression that the survival time of the patient cannot be significantly prolonged, either by surgery, or by succeeding therapies such as radiation or chemotherapy. Today we have indications that, even in epithelial tumors, chemotherapy has a therapeutic effect only in a few cases, and that the survival period is in fact not lengthened.

In my view, the only parameter that a therapy can be measured by is a survival period which includes a true quality of life. It is not important that a patient shows reduced tumor manifestation if this is not directly connected to lengthened survival time.

The problems related to side effects have increased and a great number of patients leave their primary and secondary oncological therapy to turn to complementary and alternative methods of treatment.

I want to emphasize the important contribution medicine can make if extended according to anthroposophical principles and, more particularly, the contribution mistletoe therapy can make to contemporary oncology.

Anthroposophically extended medicine is not an alternative. It can only truly be effective if it incorporates the medicine of natural science, as well as other complementary forms of therapy and medicine.

General Questions

What are the causes of cancer?

There are many causes for the appearance of cancer. Today we know that the development of cancer occurs in several stages, and that the foundation for such an illness can be laid as early as childhood. It has been determined that cancer patients often lacked "nest warmth" in childhood; in other words that these people often had to do without maternal nurturing.

During childhood, creativity should be fostered and developed through education. Children should be given a healthy daily rhythm and, in their home environment through the mood prevailing there, learn to distinguish between right and wrong. Children must be encouraged to develop their particular abilities and personalities so they can later meet the challenges life offers them.

During the adult years there are many factors that can trigger the appearance of cancer.

First, there are the physical carcinogens, for example in cigarettes. Then there is what I call an arrhythmical lifestyle—lacking a regular routine of proper nutrition, sleep, and relaxation. This often leads to regulatory disorders on a cellular level that, after a while, are hard to reverse. Rhythmic disturbances, triggered by influences such as hormone therapy, excessive food intake, sleeping pills and other synthetic medications lead to pre-cancerous conditions or cancers.

In conclusion, cancer often begins in early childhood or youth with a disturbance on the spiritual–emotional level—that level which plays a guiding role in relation to life and physical body. Stressful situations and life crises, as well as illnesses caused by excessive consumption of refined foods, alcohol, and synthetic medication, have the same effect. This results not only in an overall weakening of the immune system, but a certain inner "blindness" towards harmful influences. If control lapses in a part of the body which is already so predisposed, the cells in that area experience an emancipation. In other words, a malignant tumor can develop.

The weakening of the body's formative energies on the one hand, and harmful influences of the contemporary environment on the other, lead to the cancer process already described. This process begins on the mental-emotional level of the human being, and slowly invades the entire physical body.

Is cancer really an illness of our time?

If we take a look at the history of medicine, we can see that every century has had its own unique challenges in the form of one or another severe and far-reaching illness. Some centuries witnessed the devastating consequences of contagious diseases such as bubonic plague and cholera. In more recent times, tuberculosis has claimed many lives.

Today, the impression that cancer is increasing dramatically is not merely apparent through modern diagnosis. More tumor illnesses are being discovered in a greater number of people; a proportionately greater number of the world population is actually being diagnosed with the disease.

Is cancer limited to a particular age group?

In the past, some types of cancer appeared only in particular age groups. Testicular cancer, for example, appeared primarily in men aged thirty to thirty-five, while prostate cancer was usually was detected in men sixty years or older. Today things have changed. Physicians now encounter patients who develop testicular cancer at eighty, and others who develop prostate cancer at thirty-five. Apparently cancer is developing in a more chaotic way. Sometimes cancer in the primary phase already appears with metastases, bypassing the usual period of latency.

Is cancer becoming more aggressive?

We encounter growing numbers of patients in our practice who, already at the diagnostic stage of the illness, have metastases in life-threatening areas, such as liver or lungs. We have the impression that, in addition to the increasingly chaotic nature of cancer, its aggressiveness has also markedly increased.

How does increased aggressiveness of the carcinoma affect treatment with Iscador?

With many cancer patients, a physician does not have time to choose the right therapy at leisure. In order to establish the mistletoe therapy best suited to the individual patient, a trial period is needed. Previously, physicians had far more time to choose the right preparation following surgery, studying its effects on a patient. Today there are increasing numbers of cancer patients for whom there is only one chance to find the correct preparation. Because of the speedy progression of the illness, the therapy simply *must* work; there is no second chance. This is especially true of pancreatic and metastasizing cancers.

Is cancer treatment completed once surgery and subsequent therapies such as radiation or chemotherapy have been administered?

In my opinion, real therapy only starts once primary therapy has been concluded. By primary therapy we mean surgery and its subsequent therapies, such as chemotherapy or radiation, depending of course on both the stage the cancer is at and the type of tumor it is. Certainly these primary therapies are often necessary. However, they only serve to eliminate the tumor and other possible tumor manifestations. Contemporary clinical diagnosis cannot, however, detect micrometastases. Many of these therapies are carried out simply because of the suspicion that there might already be micrometastases in the rest of the body, as in breast cancer, where a lymph node might be affected. Whether this form of treatment is successful is often questionable. If it were to succeed in every case, no further metastasis would occur. Furthermore, these primary therapies deal only with the physical manifestations of cancer. They do not consider the circumstances that led to the cancer. In my opinion, it is essential that the *causes* of cancer also be treated, and not only the physical manifestations of the disease.

What symptoms make possible the early detection of cancer?

First, closely observe bodily eliminations, for example abnormal or unexpected bleeding, which should always be investigated. Furthermore, carefully monitor and inspect any changes in the skin. By observing the whole person, one can usually determine if the subject is a "pre-cancerous" type, with a predisposition to the disease. In patient case histories, note especially any lack of childhood illnesses, especially when no febrile conditions were obtained. Sleep disturbances, digestive and liver functional disturbances with intolerance to certain foods, and episodes of constipation should be investigated, as well as hormonal disturbances, fatigue and very slow recovery from illness.

On an emotional level, you should look for depression, for difficulty in coming to terms with problems or expressing feelings, and difficulty in establishing contact with the environment, as well as lack of interest, lack of initiative, and lack of self-confidence. Of course, it is hard to connect these symptoms with cancerous illnesses. Fatigue is a symptom of many other illnesses. Nevertheless, it is important to keep cancer in mind simply because those involved might not recognize what has been building up over a long time.

Questions About the History of Mistletoe Therapy

What is mistletoe?
Mistletoe is a semi-parasite that lives on other plants, mostly trees and bushes. It draws water and mineral salts from its host, but is capable of photosynthesis in order to manufacture its own carbohydrates. There are several hundred of types of mistletoe in the world, mostly in tropical and sub-tropical climates. They differ in form, leaf, blossom and fruit.

The Europe mistletoe is an evergreen with white berries (*Viscum album*). Botanically, it encompasses three types, growing on different types of trees: deciduous, fir, and pine mistletoe.

Mistletoe has its own growth rhythm. The berries ripen in November or December and are consumed by birds, mostly a kind of thrush. The seeds rapidly pass through the bird's intestines, and are eliminated on the branches of trees, where they stick. These seeds need light for their further development. Without light they lose their ability to germinate. Once germinated, they penetrate into the bark of the branch, as far as the cambium.

Mistletoe grows very slowly. The first tiny leaves appear in the second summer, the buds in the fifth to sixth year. The plant will not bear fruit until the end of the sixth or seventh year. And it takes seventeen months from the beginning of flower formation to the ripened berries, while a plant such as the rose needs only five months.

Since when has therapy with mistletoe been known?

Mistletoe was known in ancient times. In the sixth book of his *Aeneid,*Virgil describes how Aeneas, with the help of a golden twig similar to mistletoe, crosses through the underworld unharmed. Further mentions of mistletoe are found in a description by Pliny and in the ancient Nordic song cycle, the *Edda.* The ancient druids had a fundamental knowledge of medicine and healing. They venerated mistletoe and it was one of their universal remedies.

In the Middle Ages mistletoe was used in a variety of complaints, such as epilepsy, high blood pressure, stenocardia, asthma, sterility, depression, and sleep disorders. In some folklore it possessed mystical properties; supposedly protecting against fire and illness, ensuring a happy marriage for engaged couples, and bringing good luck.

Has mistletoe always been used for the treatment of cancer?
Only through the indications of Rudolf Steiner did it become known that mistletoe could be used to treat cancer. It was first developed as an injection in the earlier part of the last century, whereas in the Middle Ages it was administered in liquid form or as a tea.

How is the mistletoe plant made into medicine?
Mistletoe is harvested from different host trees such as apple, oak, and pine. The mistletoe used in the preparation of Iscador is harvested twice a year, in June and in November/December. The juice is extracted through a special process. Then summer and winter juices are mixed together. This ensures that preparation contains extracts from all stages of the growth cycle, leaves, stalks, berries, seeds, and flowers. A special centrifuge processes the tincture further, and a different preparation is made from each tree type of mistletoe.

Mistletoe as a Medicinal Plant

Since when has mistletoe been investigated experimentally?
In 1906, Gaultier published a work on the blood pressure lowering effects of mistletoe. In 1930, Kaelin published a study on the treatment of cancer with Viscum. These works were the starting point for various investigators who further explored mistletoe therapies. In 1932, Madaus showed that application of freshly crushed mistletoe paste on a fresh wound prevented the wound from healing, by retarding cell multiplication. In 1936, Havas published results of a study showing the effects of mistletoe extracts on the growth of plant tumors.

Koch found in 1938 that surface tumors in animals became necrotic when mistletoe was injected into and around them. The product Plenosol was developed from these experiments. In 1954, the Russian researcher Chernov published a paper about the efficacy of mistletoe in tumors near the surface of the skin. Buhl showed the efficacy of Iscador in mice with tumors, where mice treated with Iscador lived longer than control mice. In 1961, Müller showed a polysaccharide with a strong tumor inhibiting effect. Vester identified a mistletoe protein complex in 1968 that had the highest tumor inhibiting and cytostatic effect to date. Franz and Luther showed the tumor inhibiting and immune stimulating effects of mistletoe lectins between 1975 and 1985. Khwaja could positively influence the survival time of tumor-carrying mice through alkaloid-like mistletoe substances in 1980. Since then, mistletoe research has become very extensive.

What substances does mistletoe contain?
Mistletoe contains viscotoxins, lectins and the so-called Vester's proteins, as well as amino acids, alkaloids, polysaccharides, and vitamin C.

What are viscotoxins?
Viscotoxins are a group of at least five different proteins with basic characteristics, which show a cytotoxic, or cell poisoning, effect in a cell culture. Viscotoxins can attach themselves to nucleic acids, and are amazingly heat resistant. They are toxic, resulting in cell death from high doses. In weaker doses in animal tests, hypertension, bradycardia, and a negative-inotropic effect on the heart muscle were observed. The growth of human tumor cells becomes significantly inhibited.

What are lectins?
Lectins consist of a large group of substances found in most living beings. They are types of protein, which can specifically recognize and reversibly affix themselves to particular free and cell-membrane-bound sugar types. Characteristically, lectins agglutinate the cells to which they affix, for example erythrocytes, lymphocytes, or malignant cells. This can result in a toxic or hormone-like effect, even with very weak doses.

The first lectins in mistletoe were observed in 1956. In the meantime, further lectins have been discovered. Mistletoe lectin I appears most frequently and is the most cytotoxic. A total molecule of mistletoe lectin I has a strong cytotoxic effect on cell cultures. It also stimulates the immunological character of certain cells, thereby causing an increase in lymphocytes, and allowing verification of immunomodulating characteristics.

What can be said about the other constituents of mistletoe?
Vester's proteins are toxic for tumor cells, and have a cytostatic effect. They also lead to thymus enlargement, which has been verified by various investigations. *Alkaloids* are also toxic for tumor cells, but their importance is not yet clear. *Polysaccharides* may have an immune boosting effect, from the stimulation of the neutrophil granulocytes. *Amino acids*, such as arginine, are related to immune stimulation and thymus enlargement. *Vitamin C* found in mistletoe may also be immune stimulating. As a whole, mistletoe contains a rich mix of effective substances, and to these are added further substances arising during the preparation and fermentation processes.

What Iscador preparations are available?
Iscador (also called Iscar in the US) preparations from the following host trees are available:
a) *Viscum mali* (apple tree mistletoe)—Iscar M
b) *Viscum pini* (pine mistletoe)—Iscar P
c) *Viscum quercus* (oak mistletoe)—Iscar Qu

Why are mistletoe plants from different host trees used?
Rudolf Steiner, who first suggested using mistletoe in the treatment of cancer, gave indications for the use of mistletoe plants from different host trees in the treatment of different tumor types. Other empirical findings have subsequently been added. Today, gas chromatography and other mistletoe content analy-

ses can verify that especially the apple and oak mistletoe types are quite different, with different substances.

Clinical Application of Mistletoe Therapy

What results can one observe using mistletoe therapy?

Regarding immune stimulation there is a clear increase in the body's natural immunity. Many patients report a change in their warmth organism in the sense that they no longer feel cold; they sometimes manifest a slight feverish condition. There is improvement in the general feeling of well being and productivity. Appetite and sleep improve, even when the tumor cannot be reduced, or a further spreading of the tumor cannot be prevented. A definite lessening of tumor-related pain can also be observed. The main effect, however, is the inhibition of malignant growth, which is achieved without affecting healthy tissue.

Can metastases be treated?

Malignant primary tumors as well as metastases are the domain of Iscador treatment, which is often successful in preventing or stabilizing the spread of metastases. Every patient wants metastases to disappear. However, this can be an unrealistic wish. Patients nevertheless often live longer with Iscador treatment. Extensive conventional therapy may reduce the size or number of metastases, but taxes the patient's immune system to the point where there is often no strength left to fight an advancing tumor, or to increase survival time.

What are some known side effects of mistletoe?
One known side effect is the slight rise in body temperature, which is actually a desired effect. At the injection site, patients may also experience a slight inflammatory reaction, but this usually only appears with higher concentrations. It is not an allergic reaction.

Can or should one do anything about the inflammation?
The inflammation at the injection site should be left alone, unless the patient is in great discomfort. In that case, simply apply compresses of Weleda *Calendula Essence*, Weleda *Arnica Essence* or *Mercurialis perennis* ten percent ointment. In the case of pruritus (itching) *Combudoron Lotion* compresses have been helpful.

Can Iscador be administered at the same time as chemotherapy?
Treatment with Iscador can and should be administered during chemotherapy, since the latter causes a decrease in the white blood cell count. Iscador has a stabilizing effect on this. The dosage will possibly have to be increased during chemotherapy in order to more strongly stimulate the patient's immune system. Need for this must be determined individually by the physician. Generally, tolerance to chemotherapy is improved by simultaneous treatment with *Iscador*.

Can Iscador be administered in conjunction with hormone therapy?

Iscador can be administered in conjunction with all hormone treatments, both oral medications and subcutaneous or intramuscular injections. Because hormone therapies tend to disturb rhythm and decrease temperature, the use of Iscador is recommended. Care should be taken not to inject Iscador near hormone implants.

Can Iscador be administered during radiation therapy?

Yes, but not into the actual area being radiated. The injection should be at least one hand's breadth away from the area of radiation. Radiation therapy also has an immune depressing effect on the patient, which makes therapy with Iscador essential. The side effects of radiation, including excessive fatigue, can be lessened by its use.

How should therapy with Iscador be administered?

There are two phases of therapy: the induction phase and the maintenance phase. During the induction phase it is important to assess the reaction of the patient to Iscador in order to avoid an initial reaction. Therefore, it is advisable to begin with a weak preparation. The course of events during the maintenance phase depends on the condition of the patient: what other therapies are being administered (e.g. chemotherapy or radiation therapy) and to what degree the cancer has spread. During the induction phase it is always good to begin with a 0.01 mg dosage, increasing this very gradually until the proper individual dosage has been achieved.

What type of patient reactions can be expected?
The individual reaction to dosage can be assessed by:
1. The improvement of general well-being and lessening of tumor-related pain;
2. Temperature reactions, in the sense of a (desired) slight increase in body temperature;
3. Improvement of immunological status, which can be documented as an increase in the T helper cells and a reduction in the T suppressor cells, as well as an increase in the eosinophils and the absolute lymphocyte count;
4. Local inflammatory reactions up to a maximum of inches inches in diameter.

What improvements in well-being can be achieved?
1. Improvement in well being include an increase in appetite and weight, a normalization of sleep patterns, a feeling of warmth, increased productivity, and a psychological improvement.
2. Many patients show an increased lust for life with the treatment, as well as improved social integration.
3. A decrease in tumor-related pain can also be expected, and painkilling medication can be dramatically decreased.

Is it important to measure temperature?
In the early phase of mistletoe therapy, temperature is the only reaction, besides the local skin response. Measuring temperature is meaningful only if it is done before begin of the treatment, and then first thing every morning, and every evening around 6 pm, after resting for half an hour. If the rest period is

not adhered to, a change in temperature may bear no relation to Iscador. Physiologically, evening temperature is usually slightly higher than morning temperature. The increase must be at least 0.9 degrees Fahrenheit to ascertain a true temperature increase rather than one merely related to physiological activity. Remember that most painkillers lower temperature, as do hormonal preparations.

Today, in my opinion, measuring temperature has less meaning. It is now possible to measure the immunological phenomena in the patient before and after therapy, which has more value than temperature indicators ever had.

If a patient is scheduled for surgery, should mistletoe therapy begin earlier?
It is highly desirable that patients receive two series of Iscador before surgery, as this stimulates the immune system. The operation can sometimes trigger a spread of malignant cells. This may happen especially in the case of tumors that cannot be fully removed.

Is it advisable to postpone the operation for four weeks so that a course of Iscador injections can be administered?
That is an individual decision. One should bear in mind that breast cancer may already have been developing for two or three years before its clinical discovery. It is, therefore, meaningless that some physicians fall into a state of panic and schedule an operation for the next day, in cases where a long development period can be assumed. The operation should, however, not be postponed for long, because of the tendency for metastases. I

would advise at least one series of Iscador injections before surgery (fourteen days). However, it is up to each individual and their physician to decide whether he or she can postpone surgery for their particular type of cancer, or with the knowledge of having cancer.

How long should Iscador therapy be administered in cases of breast cancer?

Because these often metastasize late, a long period of therapy is advisable. The minimum treatment period, I would say, is five years. In the fifth year, if there has been no metastasis and the immune status is favorable, only seven series of Iscador injections need be given. The prescribing physician should decide whether there are risk factors that require an increased period of therapy.

Are there cancers that have to be treated with Iscador throughout a patient's life?

As soon as a metastasis occurs, therapy with Iscador should not be stopped. The patient's response to treatment has to be continuously monitored, and possibly the host tree or dosage changed. In malignant melanomas, skin and organ metastases have been described after a lapse of forty years. Therefore therapy should be continued for more than twenty or thirty years, and the frequency of therapy individually determined.

Which types of tumors react well to Iscador?

Studies show a significant increase in patient survival time with treatment of Iscador in various stages of cervical, ovarian, vaginal, mammary, stomach, bronchial, and other carcinomas, all of which indicate the efficacy of Iscador treatment.

Questions About Administering Mistletoe Therapy

How should one inject?

Injections should be subcutaneous, which is under the skin, at an angle of forty-five degrees. Many people inject too superficially; in other words showing a slight bump on the surface of the skin after the injection has been given. Then the injection is too much in the region of the hypodermis with its sensitive nerves, resulting in increased pain and possible allergic reactions.

What is the usual length of time for injection therapy?

With most types of tumor, eighty percent of relapses and metastases appear during the first two years after primary therapy. It is, therefore, absolutely necessary for Iscador to be administered for at least two years. After this, the administering physician should decide whether to introduce longer pauses between the injection series. It depends on individual state of health, tumor size, and the risk of possible metastasis.

Are there critical phases in mistletoe therapy?

Critical phases in mistletoe therapy appear especially in conjunction with immunosuppressive therapies such as chemotherapy, radiation therapy, and hormone therapy. In such cases, monitoring should be done more frequently and therapy should be adjusted according to the immune status of the patient. At times when a patient's emotions or body are more greatly stressed—viral infection is an example—treatment should be intensified. In the case of loss of employment or other strokes of destiny that are not overcome, therapy should be intensified. It is important that the treating doctor has detailed knowledge of the patient's circumstances in order to be able to assess the existing risks.

How often is Iscador usually injected?

As a rule Iscador is injected three times a week. After every four-teen injections there is a week's pause. In the case of severe risk to the patient, an injection can be given every second day, with a three-day pause after the seventh injection. When the course of injections is satisfactory, the pauses can gradually be increased. A one-week pause could be extended to two weeks in the second year, then to three or four weeks in the third year of treatment. Treatment should not, however, go below ten series (seven ampules each) per year. In special cases it may also make sense to administer Iscador daily without any pauses, as in the case of an advanced illness. However, if the dosage is increased to that intensity, regular monitoring must be done to avoid over-stimulation.

Can one inject oneself with Iscador?

It is often asked whether patients can carry out therapy at home or if it is necessary to come to the medical office. There are dif-ferent viewpoints on the issue. For some it is impossible to visit the medical office every second day or three times a week. For others it is necessary, in order to experience the therapeutic interaction with the physician. Each patient must make the decision to either carry out the therapy at home or with the help of the physician. In most cases, at-home injection therapy has proven successful, with the patient coming in for regular monitoring. When injecting at home, it is important that the patient rest afterward. When receiving injections at the medical office, the trip is frequently combined with shopping or other activities, which does not enhance the absorption of the remedy.

Should one inject in the morning or in the evening?
Because injections should be administered during the ascending temperature curve, they optimally take place before ten in the morning. Many patients, however, are very restless in the morning. For example, parents with cancer may be busy in the morning with spouses and children. If the parent cannot find the tranquillity needed for an early morning injection it is better to inject in the evening when it is peaceful, and then to have a long period of rest afterwards.

Experience in my practice has shown that one cannot assume that evening injections are less efficacious. Much more important is the period of rest afterwards, which should be about half an hour in duration.

Are there special "tricks" for administering the injection?
The injection site should be close to the tumor or to the endangered area. The distance should be one to two inches (three centimeters) from a tumor and at least four inches (ten centime-

ters) from a malignant melanoma. This is only true for existing cancers that could not be removed by surgery. For all other cancers one can assume injecting where it is most practical, although not always advisable at the site of operation, because scarring or lymphostasis can hinder absorption.

We recommend that the injection be administered in the abdomen. Taking the belly button as the middle point of a circle, the patient should inject, a hand's breadth from the belly button, around the center. The skirt or trousers waistband area should, however, be avoided, to prevent local irritation. The thigh can be used as an alternative. The upper arm, especially in the case of operated breast cancer, ought to be avoided if possible.

Can Iscador be administered intravenously?

Only experienced therapists should administer an infusion therapy with Iscador. This may be recommended in cases of increased tumor pain or when an advanced cancer cannot be arrested with normal injection therapy. Another indication for mistletoe infusion is very low immunity, which, despite increases in therapy or a change to another kind of Iscador, does not be improve.

There are particular guidelines for Iscador infusion, which will not be discussed further here, because they are strictly for use by experienced therapists. A strong allergic reaction should always be expected in the case of an infusion, and therefore the administering physician should be prepared for emergency treatment.

Questions About Immunology

What is to be understood by the regulation of immunity?
The primary purpose of the immune system is to ensure the health, integrity, and individual nature of the living organism. Without its good health, the body cannot protect itself from foreign information carriers, and positive development—continued growth—would be impossible. Evolution presupposes differences between individuals; these differences are maintained throughout life by means of an active immune system. In this context, the regulation of immunological recognition and of defense mechanisms is of central importance.

There are two areas of immunological regulation. The autoimmune system includes all influences generated within the immune system itself. Regulatory influences, such as hormonal or central nervous system activity arising in the pituitary gland, influence the immune system from other systems in the body.

Immune regulatory mechanisms become understandable through the developmental history of participating cells. These can all be traced back to a hematopoietic stem cell, and develop specific functions by means of differentiation. Cell differentiation, their multiplication, and their functional actions are regulated by many factors, often including a feedback mechanism that prevents over-reaction. Most interesting are the macrophages, the killer cells and B cells, which group themselves around granulocytes and mast cells. Their interactions are regulated by cytokines, which are very differentiated.

What can be understood by immunological status?

Improved immunological status means an increase in leukocytes and a change in concentration of the individual leukocyte sub-populations. An increase of granulocytes can be noted, especially those of eosinophils. The immune system is very disharmonious in most cancer patients; the T helper cells are exhausted; the T8 suppressor cells are massively increased; and the natural killer cells, which can directly destroy tumor cells, have been massively decreased. A harmonization in this area indicates an improvement of the immunological status.

What influence do emotions have on immune status?

A new branch of research, called psychoneuroimmunology, has recently been developed. This science shows that the brain participates in immune regulation. It has been acknowledged for decades that strokes of destiny that cannot fully be overcome or clinically depressive states have a direct influence on the immune system. Today, this can be demonstrated and verified by examining nerve activity.

What tests are used to determine immune status?

Immune status is based primarily on the differentiation of immune-competent killer cells. The so-called T helper cells and the T suppressor cells are of special clinical interest, as are the natural killer cells, which can have a direct effect on tumor cells.

Where can such an immune status test be carried out?

An analysis of immune competent cells can be carried out in every laboratory with the necessary facilities. Any physician can send a patient's blood sample to such a laboratory for an immune status test.

What are T helper cells?

T helper cells (characterized by the surface antigens T4) are understood to be cells that can recognize an antigen presented by a macrophage. T helper cells also activate B cells to form antibodies via plasma cells, activate T8 (suppressor) cells, and activate macrophages to phagocytosis.

What are suppressor cells?

Suppressor cells, distinguished by the surface marker T8, recognize and dissolve target cells, the presence of which are indicated by helper cells. They also suppress immune responses, which counteract hyperimmunity, as well as maintaining individual tolerance, together with the helper cells.

What is a lymphocyte transformation test?

The lymphocyte transformation test determines whether immune cells are immunologically competent. Frequently, immunologically competent cells multiply due to unspecific stimuli or medications. In other words, we can observe an increase of lymphocytes and T helper cells, along with a decrease of T suppressor cells. It is necessary to determine whether these cells are really active—that is whether they can recognize tumor cells and engage in anti-tumor activity.

The lymphocyte transformation test indicates whether activity is indeed possible, not only by counting the cells, but also by determining the development of aggressiveness in these cells. This test should be performed at regular intervals in order to establish whether cell counts achieved by the therapy are immunologically competent.

What clinical significance does immune status have?

Determining relative and absolute quantities of lymphocyte subpopulations is not only meaningful for the diagnosis of immunological illnesses, but also for therapy. Defects in the defense system, determined by the shift of concentrations within the lymphocyte subpopulation, can be diagnosed with this method. Regular monitoring during treatment enables the physician to draw further conclusions from the parameters of the findings. Immune suppression is a notable symptom of tumor illnesses and is often indicated by an increase in T suppressor cells, a decrease in T helper cells, and a relatively low number of natural killer cells. Immune suppression is often present after chemotherapy, radiation, or cortisone treatment. However, such changes are also frequently observed before clinical diagnosis of a tumor.

Displacement of absolute cell counts in the lymphocyte subpopulation can occur frequently, especially after chemotherapy or radiation, when there is not only a decrease in the total leukocyte count, but a decrease in the absolute lymphocyte subpopulation as well.

What immunological results are known in treatment with Iscador?

Effects on thymus and spleen have been described in animal and other studies, stimulation of the T lymphocytes and harmonization of the various lymphocyte subpopulations. Investigations have shown an effect on B lymphocytes—in other words, on the humoral immune reaction. The effects on total lymphocyte counts, neutrophils, and eosinophils has also been described. The influence on the activity of granulocytes and the activity of macrophages has also been investigated, as has been the effect on basophils and mast cells.

Furthermore, there are investigations concerning the so-called peritumoral reactivity of the organism, which concerns the change of the tissue around the tumor, where clearly discernable inflammatory infiltrations can be positively evaluated.

How effective is Iscador in terms of immunological parameters?

Many studies prove conclusively that Iscador increases the immune cell count, which includes the total lymphocyte count and granulocyte count. This leads to improved immune competence. Iscador has a regulating effect by redirecting displaced immune cells to their regulatory function. The cytokines regulate the stimulation or inhibition of various cells involved in immune reaction; their efficiency increases with Iscador treatment. One can assume that Iscador has a stimulating and harmonizing effect on many cytokines. Iscador also regulates overstimulation, a possible result of tumor-related factors. Generally, Iscador increases the immunological competence of the organism, so that the tumors are recognized as an enemy, and the dissolution of tumor cells can begin. Often the tumor is masked, which means it can no longer be recognized as such by the immune cells.

What are natural killer cells?

As the name suggests, natural killer cells have an important function in fighting tumors. In terms of developmental history, natural killer cells are older than T lymphocytes. They also regulate B cell differentiation and hematopoiesis, or blood formation.

What are macrophages?

Macrophages are the cells that provide the antigens that sensitize T cells. They play an important role in the cellular fight against viruses and tumors, destroying viruses and tumor cells by means of chemotaxis, enzymes, or phagocytosis.

What are B lymphocytes?

B lymphocytes are plasma cells that produce antibodies. They are stimulated by antigens or degenerated cells. These cells serve as a defense against infections, and produce antibodies as a result of the antigen stimulus of tumor cells.

What are circulating immune complexes?

Circulating immune complexes come into existence as a result of the reaction of an antibody to an antigen. Antibodies are produced in tumor patients as a reaction against tumor cells. These tumorassociated antibodies can, together with corresponding antigen substances, create circulating immune complexes. At a certain concentration level, these immune complexes are no longer disturbed by macrophages. They then gather around the tumor creating a barrier that prevents an active immunological reaction against the tumor cells. They also block the macrophage function, immobilizing any effective defense mechanism against tumor cells.

Results of Treatment with Iscador

Are there clinical results for therapy with mistletoe?

There are many clinical studies on the treatment of various tumors with Iscador. These are mostly retrospective studies, but there are also prospective, randomized studies. In retrospective studies an analysis is made a few years after therapy, and the efficacy of the treatment is compared to data in established literature. In prospective, randomized studies a study goal is determined, therapy is established, and the patient is randomly assigned to a group. Neither the physician nor the patient know whether the treatment is active or a placebo.

Based on many years of experience, anthroposophical doctors are convinced of the efficacy of treatment with Iscador, and feel that it is unethical to withhold mistletoe therapy from patients. For them it is out of the question that a patient who wants Iscador should be refused treatment, or be subjected to randomization. This reduces the possibility of carrying out randomized, prospective studies.

Are randomized prospective studies necessary?

In my opinion such studies are not necessary, because ethically they can only be carried out with great difficulty. It makes far more sense to observe well-documented individual cases. This is done by creating so-called "matched pairs," which means finding patients with the same course of illness and the same starting point, and to document these cases.

A well-documented individual course of illness says far more about the curative possibilities of a preparation than large statistics in which many patients have to be excluded because of detailed rules. Most conventional medicine in use today was tested retrospectively.

What research has been done for breast cancer in women?
Three studies were carried out at the Lukas Clinic in Arlesheim, Switzerland. In a retrospective study of 319 women, more were alive ten years later who had received adequate treatment with Iscador than those who received inadequate Iscador treatment. Inadequate treatment is defined as the family physician deciding independently not to continue a patient's Iscador treatment. The percentages were sixty-five percent compared to thirty-eight percent for clinical stage I (breast cancer without lymph nodes affected) and thirty-three percent compared to seventeen percent for stage II (breast cancer with lymph nodes effected).

A second study made an historical comparison between patients receiving adequate treatment over a long time compared to those who broke off treatment with Iscador after a short time. The average survival time for patients who received adequate treatment with Iscador was nearly twice as long as for those who did not receive adequate treatment.

A third retrospective study, also involving recurrent and metastasizing late stages, showed similar results. The effectiveness of Iscador treatment in breast cancer patients is clear in practice. Many of my own patients have profited from treatment with Iscador, and are living longer with metastases than they would have without treatment.

What other studies are available?

Further studies have been done on ovarian carcinomas, cervical, colon. and rectal cancers, and on bladder cancer. There are also studies available on lung, stomach, and skin cancer, and on pleural carcinomatosis. The common element in all these studies is that patients treated with Iscador live longer. In studies where well being is central, a definite increase in well being was observed, especially in comparison to other therapies.

Recently there have been warnings about therapy with Iscador. What is the background to this?

More information about the immune system is now available. For example, with Iscador therapy, immune stimulating substances, including cytokines, are produced. Lately, one has also found so-called cytokine receptors in different types of cancer, for example ovarian and kidney carcinomas, as well as other types of tumors.

The question is whether the increased cytokine production with Iscador treatment results in the stimulation of malignant cells. Such results have not been noted in practice, nor in the studies mentioned above, nor in the anthroposophical clinics in which many of the studies have been conducted. In fact, many patients treated for ovarian cancer showed longer survival periods than has been proven possible by means of chemotherapy. Patients for whom conventional medicine had failed showed a longer survival period than literature and statistics record. Therefore, there is absolutely no evidence that stimulation of malignant cells occurs as a result of mistletoe therapy.

As recent investigations show, mistletoe preparations have a harmonizing effect on cytokines. This means that cytokine fractions, decreased as a result of the tumor illness, clearly increased, while on the other hand the excess of excreted cytokines returned to normal.

One can assume that improved immunological competence can be achieved by means of mistletoe therapy, and that stimulation resulting from the harmonizing process seems not to be likely.

What are the results with malignant melanomas?

Malignant melanomas belong to a group of tumors that react very well to immunomodulatory therapies. Trials in earlier years regarding immune stimulation with other medications, such as *BCG,* have already been completed.

A study done at the dermatology department of the University Clinic in Basel, Switzerland, shows clearly that patients survive longer after treatment with Iscador. This study is underscored by other observations. A study on melanoma patients was carried out in my own practice. This study resulted in evidence across the board of a prolonged survival period. And in the case of three patients, there was even a regression of metastases. In this situation individualized treatment, not schematic treatment as carried out in randomized studies, is important. All patients were treated individually according to their immune state, which is of primary importance for patients with malignant melanomas.

Concurrent Therapies—Medicinal

*Note: the following anthroposophical/homeopathic preparation sugges-
tions are for the prescribing physician and available from Weleda.*

Is other therapy concurrent with Iscador of value?

Therapy concurrent with Iscador is meaningful in the case of
tumor localizations or metastases, or in the case of general
cancer symptoms. There are, for example, particular medicines
for hemostasis, effusions, febrile conditions, bone metastases,
and for regulating circulation and intestinal function. Analgesic
medication for acute or chronic pain may be required. Skin
reactions to radiation should also be treated.

What concurrent therapy can be used in the case of bone metastases?

Homeopathic medicines may be chosen by the physician in
conjunction with Iscador treatment, for example an ampule of
Cerussite 8X every day or every second day, combined with
Pyromorphite 8X or *Fluorite 6X* as a subcutaneous injection.
These preparations have been shown to be effective against pain
and for the stimulation of bone formation.

What other concurrent therapies are meaningful for the treatment of pain?

Iscador has a painkilling effect and may enable a reduction of
analgesics. For severe pain, Iscador infusions may be considered.
Different kinds of tumor pain have benefited from the following treatment:

1. *Formica 3X/Formica 15X AA amp*: daily one ampule subcutaneously.
2. *Apis/Rhus toxicodendron comp.*: daily one ampule subcutaneously.

In the case of chronic pain conditions, one to two ampules of *Aurum 30X/Equisetum arvense 20X AA* can be injected subcutaneously daily. In the case of nerve pain the preparation *Naja comp.* has proven effective. One to two ampules can be injected daily, subcutaneously.

Is there a remedy for a skin reaction to radiation?

Weleda *Skin Tonic* and *Lotio pruni comp. cum Cupro* have proven to be effective in the treatment of this condition. These remedies should be applied frequently to the radiated areas to prevent skin reactions. They are also effective for the prevention of bedsores. Daily application of *Quartz 1% Oil* in the area of an operation or radiation has also proven to be beneficial. In the case of skin reactions to radiation, *Combudoron Liquid or Weleda Burn Care* is recommended as a daily application.

Is there a therapy for ulcerated tumors?

Calendula Ointment 10%, Viscum pini Gel 10% or *Viscum pini 5% Ointment* are effective in the treatment of this condition.

Is there a remedy for hemorrhaging?

To contain acute bleeding in tumor tissue *Stibium metallicum praeparatum 6X* ampules have been especially effective. Two to five 1 ml ampules or one 10 ml ampule should be administered daily. Intravenous administration has been especially effective.

In the case of abdominal bleeding *Stibium metallicum praeparatum 0.4%* suppositories are recommended. In the case of gynecological bleeding *Berberis Decoctum 3X* ampules can be injected subcutaneously once or twice daily.

What preparations can be used for the stabilization of circulation in conjunction with Iscador?

For the treatment of circulatory disturbances, which are relatively frequent in cancer patients, *Cardiodoron* is effective. Fifteen to twenty drops should be taken three times daily. *Veratrum album Decoction 4X,* twenty drops three times daily, also leads to a definite improvement in circulation.

Is liver treatment meaningful?

The liver is often severely affected in tumor patients. On the one hand, it is a large organ with a clear immune function in the reticulo-endothelial system. On the other hand, medication, either cytostatics or painkillers, must be detoxified here, often leading to an over-burdening of the liver.

Substances released in tumor breakdown are also a toxic burden on the liver. The following medications have been effective:

1. *Carduus marianus* capsules: one or two capsules three times daily.
2. *Hepatodoron* tablets: two tablets three times daily.
3. *Chelidonium/ Curcuma* tablets: one tablet three times daily.

What remedy is effective for the regulation of digestion?
Digestodoron, tablets or drops, is an effective remedy. This medication leads to a clear improvement in the secretion and mobility of the digestive tract, as well as a reduction of heartburn, nausea, bloating, and diarrhea. Fluid intake, which has a regulatory function regarding good digestion, should be increased. A medicinal therapy without adequate fluid intake does not seem to be as effective.

Concurrent Therapies—Artistic Therapies

Are artistic therapies applied concurrently with Iscador effective?
Artistic therapy presupposes an expanded understanding of illness and health when included in a treatment plan.

Cancer treatment should include the whole human being, not just the physical body. We do not only target physical well being with our various therapies; emotional and spiritual well being play as much of a role in recovery.

Artistic therapies—especially therapeutic eurythmy, therapeutic painting and sculpture, speech therapy, music therapy, and color and light therapy—serve to alleviate disturbances in the whole human being.

Is concurrent therapeutic eurythmy effective?
Therapeutic eurythmy, the need for which is always determined by the treating physician, is a specialized movement therapy conducted by a qualified eurythmist in cooperation with the prescribing physician. Through therapeutic eurythmy, cancer

patients feel that they are actively contributing to their healing process, and not merely passively at the mercy of their illness. This brings about an immediate improvement in well being.

The organic change enabled by therapeutic eurythmy cannot be detected easily by patients, because it is a long-term process. During this process the diseased organ is actually brought towards restoration of its function and form.

Eurythmy can reduce the lack of energy often experienced by cancer patients. The same is true for the loosening of rigid movement forms. Increased activity gives confidence and strength, and the courage to overcome the cancer.

Therapeutic eurythmy can reduce lymphatic congestion, reduce pain, and increase a patient's sense of inner strength, often significantly depleted. For many, it can be a strange new way of moving the body, but it brings with it the experience of previously untapped strengths and abilities. In eurythmy, emotional experience, which is ruled by the objective laws of language, is expressed in movement formation.

In my experience, the effects of curative eurythmy have been obvious. Many patients treated by us carried out this therapy with a concurrent cancer therapy, reporting that they felt better, had more courage, and experienced a decrease in many of their complaints.

What significance do artistic therapies have?

Artistic therapies should lead to a patient's sense of unity in body, soul, and spirit. One-sidedness—focussing on one of these three aspects instead of a balanced focus on all three—is, therefore, counteracted. Which artistic therapies are applicable depends on the needs of each individual patient. Therapeutic eurythmy is but one of several artistic therapies that support the patient's healing process.

Biographical Work and Related Issues

Is it significant to speak of "biographical work" in a modern context? Is this method also used as therapy?

For a long time there was no awareness of the factors in the patient's history, which often play a significant role in the development of tumors. Psychoneuroimmunology has proven that emotional experiences which have not been resolved present a great risk in the development of cancer. Patients often develop cancer after a severe emotional crisis or after a long depression. In my opinion, it is essential to include individual biographical factors when assessing the illness.

A patient with breast cancer who is supported by her husband has a much better prognosis than a patient with the same stage of cancer, who is abused by her husband because she now only has one breast. These are real examples from my practice.

Of course, it is hard for many people to examine their lives and facilitate change. Family structures are set, and change is not always possible. Family members may feel that their comfort is threatened and act accordingly. However, it is essential to discuss such factors with patients and to start an appropriate course of therapy, which may include working on oneself, showing the patient's course of life up to that point and highlighting significant, pivotal events. The patient and therapist together decide what positive changes can be made, with an emphasis on the future.

Psychotherapy is recommended only after the condition of the patient has stabilized. Psychotherapy taxes the patient heavily, because issues, suppressed for years or decades, are brought to the surface. These must be worked through, which is not possible if the patient is struggling with tumors, chemotherapy, or radiation. In such a case, speech therapy is recommended, which can, after the condition has stabilized, be carried over into psychotherapy.

Can the family help with therapy?

Family help can vary significantly depending on the situation, but is always essential regarding a change in diet, which is discussed later. It is also essential for the family to understand that tumor patients have a different concept of time.

In many cases, one must assume that, with the start of metastasis, the dying process has begun, i.e. a complete cure is no longer possible. Family support and sensitivity in accompanying the patient in this difficult process is needed. The family should not allow courage and hope to fail. Many tumor patients work for their families to the point of exhaustion, until the start of their illness. Often it is not convenient for the beneficiaries to share the work load. Many families react strongly during primary therapy and the possible subsequent chemotherapy or radiation therapy. After the conclusion of primary therapy, when the patient returns to his or her role in the family and/or the workplace, the cancer diagnosis is often forgotten and the patient becomes heavily burdened with responsibilities once again.

Obviously the return to a situation which mostly likely led to the illness in the first place is very unfavorable for the prognosis. A change in the situation could lead to healing.

Should the patient always be told the truth with regard to the prognosis?

Many studies have shown that patients can handle the truth, whereas previously this was strongly disputed. However, some people find it easier not to tell the patient the truth because they themselves don't want to face the situation. In other words, many family members—and even physicians—prefer to withhold the truth from patients so that they themselves don't have to deal with patients' normal reactions, such as despair, anger, fear, or bitterness.

This silence often leads to a situation in which both partners know the true situation but are too afraid or intimidated to discuss it with each other. The tumor patient does not want to burden his or her partner, and the partner wants to protect the patient. The result is a lack of communication, which can be a heavy burden for both in the last few months of the patient's life. This is precisely the time when patients need their families and their partner to come to terms with the patient's destiny, and to organize the things that are important to them.

Iscador in Combination
with Conventional Medicine

Can therapy with Iscador be combined with chemotherapy, hormone therapy or radiation?

In my opinion, Iscador therapy should always be carried out in conjunction with chemotherapy, radiation, or other conventional cancer treatments. During chemotherapy, the immune competence of the organism is radically reduced. Administering Iscador can provide a positive, balancing effect, which will stabilize the leukocytes. This means that chemotherapy, if necessary, can be carried out with success, and without doing greater damage to the immune system than necessary. Therapy with Iscador can often prevent the interruption of chemotherapy due to leukopenia.

Regarding surgery, injections can be administered up to the time of the operation, but should be discontinued post-operatively for fourteen days. This prevents a possible interference with wound healing or infection. After a fourteen-day break the therapy can be resumed. In the case of sensitive patients who have undergone a severe operation, a reduction in the dose may be necessary.

Does Iscador treatment work despite chemotherapy and radiation?

If a patient has been treated extensively with chemotherapy or radiation therapy, leukopenia can set in, which often remains for years. Obviously the efficacy of Iscador therapy is reduced in such a situation, because certain reaction systems have been hardened and significant results are no longer possible. However, even in such cases, it is often astonishing what can be achieved with mistletoe therapy, especially in conjunction with artistic therapy, to dissolve this hardening.

If a patient with metastases arrives for Iscador treatment after much surgery, chemotherapy, and radiation, it is not realistic to expect great results from mistletoe therapy. But, I still recommend that mistletoe therapy be started, even if only to improve the well being of the patient during the time he or she has left.

Are there special indications for treatment with Iscador in conjunction with cytostatics?

Reactions to the various cytostatics are very individualized. It is not possible to predict how severely a patient will react to a cytostatic combination. Even the new Taxol therapy, appearing initially to result in severe side effects, is tolerated by many patients, with complete hair loss being the most severe side effect.

It is not possible to predict how severely a patient is going to react to a specific combination in terms of the immunological burden. This has to be determined individually.

If a patient is to receive Interferon in conjunction with chemotherapy, should Iscador be administered anyway?

In my opinion Iscador should also be administered, but only in conjunction with immune monitoring. Chemotherapy results in severe immune deficiency, which would probably not be corrected solely by the use of Interferon. A combination of Iscador and Interferon seems promising, because of the difference in treatment for each of these therapies. The immune parameters, however, should be monitored in order to prevent overstimulation of immunity. A combination therapy that includes Interferon should not be attempted without this monitoring.

What painkillers should not be used?
Today many preparations of the *Diclofenac* type are recommended, especially for the treatment of pain in bone metastases, as in the case of prostate carcinoma. With the use of these medications it is important to know if the tumor is forming an inflammatory wall to encircle the metastases.

Studies have shown that painkillers of the *Diclofenac* type disproportionately concentrate in this inflammatory wall, thereby disturbing it. Therapy with Iscador attempts to stimulate such an inflammatory wall, and to stimulate and activate the migration of immune competent cells, such as eosinophils, into it.

Because pain therapy with *Diclofenac* preparations leads to a disturbance of this immune reaction, and is, therefore, contraindicated for therapy with Iscador, centrally working analgesics such as *Naloxone, Tramador*, or similar medications are preferred.

Success is often achieved if patients choose their own pain therapy. Many of my patients, who have learned to inject subcutaneously, have *Tramador* ampules at home. *Tramador* can also be injected subcutaneously. Patients can look after themselves very well in this way. Side effects are relatively rare, especially if the effects of the preparations have already been tested in practice.

Does hormone therapy represent a contraindication with Iscador therapy?

All hormone therapies can be administered in conjunction with mistletoe therapy. This holds true for both oral applications and implants placed under the skin of the abdomen, or administered intramuscularly by means of injections. Hormone therapy often leads to temperature rigidity, which can be balanced with mistletoe treatment, or with artistic therapies. The physical effects of hormone therapy, or the effects on sexual life, are often severe, and should be addressed by means of speech therapy.

Iscador in Combination with Alternative Medicine Approaches

Note: the following suggestions are for the prescribing physician to determine.

What methods of alternative therapy can be used in conjunction with Iscador?

So-called alternative treatments are manifold, ranging from treatment with enzyme preparations, vitamin preparations and trace elements, to ozone therapy, various kinds of blood cleansing and many alleged immune-stimulating methods. It is important to know that mistletoe therapy is not an alternative therapy, but is included within the framework of an anthroposophically extended therapy.

An anthroposophical physician who administers mistletoe is also trained in conventional medicine, and prescribes conventional therapies for the treatment of cancer. Anthroposophical doctors treat patients from a different viewpoint in the understanding of both the human being and the illness, incorporating additional medical therapies, artistic therapies, and Iscador in the treatment of cancer. Anthroposophical medicine is not an *alternative* to conventional medicine, rather an *effective enhancement* of existing, conventional therapies.

Not all alternative therapies are suited for use in conjunction with Iscador. Questionable therapies which appear to have financial gain rather than effective treatment as a goal should be avoided.

Many alternative therapies have an immune-stimulating effect, for example thymic preparations. In such cases it is important to determine if further immune stimulation is actually necessary, or whether there is a danger of overstimulation when used in combination with mistletoe therapy.

Ozone therapy can also have an immune stimulating effect, but if the wrong dosage is chosen, it can actually have an immune-depressive effect.

What about a combination therapy with vitamin A?
Stimulation of cellular and humoral immunity is possible with vitamin A treatment. An increase in antibody production has been documented with the use of vitamin A, and the development of cytotoxic T lymphocytes and an increase in the activity of natural killer cells can be observed with high dosages of vitamin A. A direct effect can also be seen in the anti-prolifer-

ating effect against the actual tumor cells. Studies have shown that bronchoscopically determined metaplasias in the bronchial mucous membrane had decreased significantly in heavy smokers with the administration of vitamin A. There are also additional studies on decreased hormone levels in the case of metaplasias in the intestinal and urogenital mucous membranes, which can be seen as the preliminaries to pre-cancerous changes.

What can be said about combination therapy with vitamin C?
Experimentally, numerous immunological reactions can be achieved with vitamin C. An extreme deficiency of this vitamin leads, among other things, to defects in cellular immunity. The most meaningful observation, however, seems to be that, with vitamin C, the transformation of amines to nitrosamines, and the amides to nitrosamides by means of nitrites, can be slowed down or prevented. In animal experiments these nitro compounds dissolve carcinomas of the liver, esophagus, stomach, kidney, and pancreas. Therefore, it makes sense to administer high doses of vitamin C in conjunction with Iscador. Vitamin C can be taken in the form of ascorbic acid powder three times a day are considered sufficient. Some patients with metastasizing tumors show that the administration of vitamin C in conjunction with infusions results in a definite stimulation in immunity.

What can be said about combination therapy with vitamin E?
Vitamin E is especially effective as an antioxidant, and is active with selenium in binding free radicals in cell membranes. These

free radicals increasingly appear in the body as a result of environmental pollution and can be a burden to the immunity of cancer patients, as well as to healthy individuals. Vitamin E, therefore, helps in the prevention of pre-cancerous conditions. Experiments prove that people with low vitamin E plasma values have a higher risk of carcinomas. This is especially true in combination with low selenium concentrations. Besides bronchial, stomach, and breast cancers, for which a significant relationship with low vitamin E plasma concentrations has been proven, colon carcinomas should also be kept in mind, although it has been difficult to prove a relationship between vitamin E levels and colon carcinomas in studies.

What about trace elements?
Trace elements play an important role in all life processes and are earning increasing importance in clinical oncology. They are used for diagnostics, and are being administered more frequently to correct deficiencies, or to achieve specific pharmacological conditions. Selenium is one of the trace elements most essential to life. About twenty years ago it was pinpointed as a possible environmental protector against cancer. Large scale experiments with selenium as a cancer preventative on risk populations are being carried out.

Selenium is a prerequisite for normal cell growth, but slower growth appears in the case of heightened concentrations, and irreversible cell damage and eventual cell death in the case of very high concentrations. Depending on the level of concentration, selenium is both a growth substance and a growth modulator, as well as a cytotoxic agent. Selenium influences the immune system. It stimulates the formation of antibodies, modulates lymphocyte proliferation, and improves the activity of macrophages and killer cells. Selenium, however, does not turn the immune activity around; dosages in high sub-toxic quantities have an immune-depressing result. Epidemiological studies show an inverse relationship between death from cancer and local selenium quantities. These findings are supported by the results of prospective studies, from which it is clear that low selenium values in healthy volunteers are an indication of the heightened risk of cancer.

In the face of these observations it is justifiable to accept the therapeutic value of selenium for tumor patients. The immunomodulatory basis of selenium is different from that of Iscador and no overlapping of the therapies occurs. A combination of selenium and Iscador, therefore, seems effective. Very high concentrations of selenium however have a cytotoxic effect.

What about therapy with zinc?
Zinc is another trace element used relatively frequently in the treatment of tumor patients. Tumor growth is influenced by changes in zinc intake; a surplus of zinc speeds the growth process, a depletion of zinc slows it down. Tumor regressions have even been observed. However, medicinal deprivation of zinc cannot be used for treating cancer in humans, due to severe side effects. Whether the cytotoxic results of chemotherapy are altered with zinc deprivation cannot be answered at this stage. An inverse relation was observed between zinc concentrations

in patients with prostate cancer and the results of therapy. Certain cytostatics results in a decrease of zinc in tumors.

Because the serum zinc values in cancer patients are mostly low, the question needs to be asked whether they will be normalized by zinc supplementation. One has to take into account that zinc can speed up tumor growth and that low zinc levels are not the result of low zinc intake, but rather the result of the tumor's need for high quantities of zinc. Zinc supplements at sub-toxic levels administered in the drinking water of mice with spontaneous mammary tumors resulted in a rapid acceleration of tumor growth. *In vivo*, zinc acted reciprocally with selenium, with the anti-cancerous results of selenium completely cancelled by zinc. This confirms the observations that there is a direct correlation between zinc intake through nourishment and the fatality of breast cancer.

We must, therefore, warn against treatment with zinc, as zinc levels necessary for therapeutic purposes are not yet known.

Is treatment with iron dangerous for tumor patients?
The role of iron in tumor development is the subject of much investigation. From such investigation it follows that iron may be essential for life, but that, in excess, it stimulates tumor growth. Excess iron is stored in the metabolically active cell membranes of tumor cells, instead of in the cytosolic ferritin as in normal cells. This enables the rapid growth of tumor cells. The iron content of tumor cells varies considerably and depends on the type of tumor. For example, breast tumors are often high in iron content.

Large quantities of iron can accumulate in tumors. In mice with large mammary tumors, the total iron content of the tumor exceeded that of the liver. Because tumor growth is dependent on iron intake, iron supplementation in anemic patients should be carefully evaluated.

For tumor prophylaxis, the same holds true for iron as it does for zinc: chronic surplus, as well as chronic deficiency, should be avoided. Resistance to cancer is decreased organ-specifically in the case of chronic iron deficiency. Iron supplementation should, as with zinc, occur via diet rather than via supplement. The absorption of both elements is especially regulated by phytic acid, which is found in wholemeal products.

What other trace elements are important in cancer therapy?
It is possible that chronic copper deficiency results in weaker resistance to cancer. Until now, copper supplements have seemed unnecessary, as copper deficiencies were observed only in rare illnesses. Chronic copper deficiency in particular is linked to bone and joint illnesses, but copper supplementation does not seem to be beneficial.

Magnesium stabilizes cell membranes, and a synergetic interaction between magnesium, selenium, and vitamin E can be assumed. It is noticeable that subnormal magnesium concentrations have been observed in almost all types of cancer, excluding melanomas. General magnesium supplements cannot however be recommended, as magnesium can accelerate tumor growth.

Nutritional Aspects

Can a specific diet be recommended for cancer patients?
There are many opinions about specific diets for cancer patients, none of which are completely convincing. Without any intake of nutrients, an existing tumor can be starved. However, all diets that aim to "starve the tumor," or, through the elimination of essential ingredients, aim to "dry out" the tumor, lead to a considerable loss of vitality in the patient, which can frequently and rapidly lead to tumor progression.

Tumor patients should follow these general nutritional criteria:

1. Use mostly fresh foods, avoid if possible preserved foods, preservatives, and artificial fertilizers.
2. Avoid alcohol. Alcohol has an inhibiting effect on the conscious higher ego, which is probably the most important aspect of the human being. Alcohol has a negative effect on the liver as well, which in our experience is the most important organ in cancer therapy.
3. Reduce the consumption of potatoes and tomatoes.
4. Seek to establish joy and rhythm in eating, and restfulness while digesting. These qualities are severely lacking in our contemporary lifestyle.

Why should tumor patients not eat potatoes?
Potatoes are not real roots, but rather stalk growths, which develop in the soil without light. If one exposes potatoes to light, they become poisonous. Cancer patients especially should avoid young potatoes, as they still have the potential to become poi-

sonous. Rudolf Steiner elaborated that potatoes belong to the group of plants known as nightshades, which burden the digestive system and can lead to dullness and general lethargy. In other words, they don't stimulate the body's restorative energies.

In experiments, the poison solanin has been found in the skin of potatoes. This poison is more evident in young potatoes, and recently the suspicion has arisen that solanin may contribute to the formation of cancer. It is important to know that in experiments on laboratory animals with tumors, the tumors grew faster in the animals fed a potato diet.

Why should tumor patients not eat tomatoes?
Rudolf Steiner explained that the tomato, according to its nature, especially stimulates that "which is independent in the organism and that which specializes." In today's medicine we know that rheumatic and gout patients should not eat tomatoes. In the case of rheumatism and gout, deposits are formed in the joints or in the muscles. One could perceive cancer as an independent deposit in the organism. We can then understand why Rudolf Steiner said that cancer patients should not eat tomatoes.

There are also animal experiments indicating that animals with tumors fed with tomatoes develop significantly larger tumors than the control group. It is furthermore important to know that tomatoes, like potatoes, also form the poison solanin.

Besides this, the unique characteristics of the tomato, such as its proliferating growth, its love of muddy ground, its ability to ripen in the dark, and the nature of the fruit to draw the last strength out of the plant in order to come to full ripeness, place the tomato in a special category. These severe characteristics are the reason why Rudolf Steiner urged cancer patients not to eat this fruit. Of course, this does not mean that tomatoes are forbidden across the board. Tomatoes can certainly be consumed by healthy individuals. It is also a misunderstanding that other nightshades should be avoided. Peppers, for example, are important nutritious plants, as are cucumbers and pumpkin-family vegetables, and should definitely be included in the tumor patient's diet.

What general guidelines should be observed in diet?
Today, along with food, the human body absorbs hundreds of different chemical substances, of which only a few serve as nutrients for the maintenance of bodily functions. Because of the possible causal link to malignant tumors, mutagenic substances in foods should be closely monitored. This includes plant additives, toxic molds that cause perishing, and mutagenic substances that can arise in the preserving, processing and preparation of ready-to-serve foods.

The likelihood that many foods could be contaminated with persistent environmental poisons, such as heavy metals, pesticides, or radioactive nuclides, all of which have mutagenic characteristics, is only mentioned here. Cancer patients should be especially careful about environmental poisons in food, but also about the possibility of foods poisoned with molds.

Molds are relatively widespread today and food contaminated with mold should generally be destroyed. Often it is not possible to see whether food is contaminated with mold spores or filaments. The mold is only visible in one place, but will have grown through the food and result in spoiling. Cancer patients suffer severely from the effects of ingesting mold.

Generally the consumption of food types that are more frequently contaminated, such as moldy nuts or highly heated, grilled pickled food, should be avoided. Food coloring should also be avoided.

Is there a link between nutrition and the immune system?
Nutrition, or individual nutrients, interact with the immune system and can inhibit or stimulate its function. Conclusions can be drawn from this for the treatment of patients with malignancies.

Different effects were found in the immune system with the intake of specific substances, such as arginine, nucleotides, and lipids. Many more tests will be necessary to determine the nutritionally induced effects on the immune system with regard to specific clinical situations, such as burns, lengthy operations, organ transplants, or tumors. However, current studies indicate promising results with immunomodulating diets.

In tests, arginine clearly influenced immunity in the human being. Furthermore, healthy volunteers who increased their daily arginine intake showed significantly increased lymphocytic reactions to mitogens. Post-operative patients, who received increased arginine by means of enteral alimentation, also showed improved lymphocytic reactions to mitogens.

In animal tests, the size and frequency of tumors could be reduced by means of increased arginine intake. Animals inoculated with a virus displayed longer latency periods regarding tumor formation and smaller tumors, when fed on an arginine-rich diet.

All studies so far indicate that arginine has an immune stimulating effect. The improved function of lymphocytes and macrophages could be important in improving post-operative immune function, and in preventing potential complications from infection. High levels of arginine can be detected in mistletoe.

Nucleotides can also influence tumor growth. In animal experiments with induced T lymphocytic tumors, the tumors were dependent on nucleotides for their full development.

Lipids are important nutrients in the reaction of the organism to nutrient deficiency and stress. It has recently been discovered that lipids, especially prostaglandins, play an important role in the immune system.

In conclusion, it can be said that immune competent cells react differently according to whether the diet contains medium chain triglycerides, omega three fatty acids and omega six fatty acids. Recent investigations show that the immune system can be influenced therapeutically and prophylactically with the administration of a special fat-containing diet. A diet can be put together in such a way that, mainly through a change in the proportion of the different kinds of fats, changes in the function of the immune system can be affected according to the need of the clinical situation.

Suggestions for Self-Help in Cancer Treatment

Erika Merz, MD

THERE ARE MANY POSSIBILITIES TO INCREASE the strength of your life forces. Creating an appropriate regimen varies in each individual case, but the crucial factor is your awareness that you are actively involved in the healing process.

- A wholesome, balanced, organic diet. It supports medication therapy through its recognized immuno-stimulating quality, and by supplementing deficiencies in trace elements and vitamins.
- Attentiveness to maintaining warmth. The goal is developing a comfortable and comforting inner warmth protection, achieved with the help of appropriate clothing (natural fibers) and physical therapy including warmth applications,

herb teas, etc. Regular, carefully applied stimulation such as alternating hot and cold foot baths can activate physiological warmth regulation and balance, and strengthen resistance to cold.

- Exercise is especially important. Spend time outdoors every day if you can. Physical activity, joyfully done, not only increases oxygen supply but creates the basis for a feeling of wellness. Consciously develop deep, relaxed breathing. This might take some instruction and practice.

- Regularity brings results! A rhythmic lifestyle is strengthening and deeply healing. Eat at the same time every day, balance activity with rest and adequate sleep. Avoid fatigue, chronic overwork, long journeys, too much sun—all known to adversely affect the immune system.

These examples are given as time-tested ways of influencing well being and vitality. They are central to the whole healing process. Discover what is possible and appropriate for your individual needs. The main point is to find a new and conscious relationship to yourself and your body—even if the latter is challenged and weakened through the illness and its treatment. By paying mindful, loving attention to your body's signals and messages, and handling yourself with care, you will create your basis for comprehensive healing.

What can I do for my soul's healing and comfort?
First and foremost, you should find help in dealing mentally with this illness. After the initial shock of the diagnosis, and the burden and isolation of invasive therapy, you should begin to

find means to bring healing, strength, and support to the soul, whose influence on the immune system is by now well recognized by doctors and researchers. Everything that nurtures inner equilibrium, hope, courage and joy must be supported, for they are important allies in the challenge of the illness.

- Of great importance is feeling embedded in a circle of people you trust. These primarily include family and friends or self-help groups, and constitute another protective layer of warmth. Or seek out supportive psychotherapy. Finding the "milieu" offering you protection, shelter, and openness, so that feelings of fear, pain, sorrow, and helplessness can be shared and carried, is important to your recovery.

- Everything that creates and enhances feelings of inner vitality, mobility, and color is deeply healing and strengthening. Colors directly nourish and support an exhausted soul, while the right music, performed or listened to intensively, invigorates and uncramps it.

- Art therapy, whether music, painting, therapeutic eurythmy, drama, dance, or sculpture is a proven tool to stimulate creative life forces. Activating the creative ability inherent in all of us is of key importance in mastering illness. Through art therapy, the disease process can be worked through; the mobilized creative forces permit a renewed feeling of unitedness with the world.

- You can develop deep powers of order and regularity by finding times of inner rest and contemplation. Create an "inner space" free of nervousness, necessity, or distraction. At first it may seem hard, even impossible, to sense the point of inner quiet in you because of constraints or lack of strength. This is just when you need to find it most. Practice proven relaxation techniques and—where possible—meditation and prayer to create the basis for inner quiet.

Your key is finding the harmonious balance between looking inward and a loving interest in the world—and a balanced rhythm of rest and activity. Both of these will help uncover new realms and sources of strength in you.

How can I seek new life goals?

Besides the assistance dealing with burdens and deepening your qualitative experience, you should find ways to inwardly reorganize and raise yourself up, cultivating those abilities in you that will give a goal and meaning to your life.

- The upheaval of the illness and its disruption of daily routine gives you a chance to step out onto new paths. Entering the unknown and finding new experiences unlock previously unknown realms of perception that allow life to be felt and grasped more consciously and more deeply than before. The illness should immediately become a "working contract" that is to bear fruit in many ways.

- In this connection it is important to find and foster in yourself those areas in which you feel most free, independent, awake, and empowered. Your goal, always within the parameters of your possibilities and personal situation, is to consciously and actively take control of your own life. This may include informing yourself about the illness and its possible treatments, and beginning an active participation in the healing process.

● Important for the activation of your inner strength potential is setting worthwhile life goals, and setting them again
and again. If you can formulate motives, ideals, and wishes
that make sense for you, and which can create enthusiasm,
you will create the basis for deep healing. This may seem a
tall order, given the many hindrances and constraints, but
practicing alertness and focus will allow you to discover and
realize which choices and decisions are most important and
make most sense. The goal is saying "yes" to your own inner
needs. The forces you unlock thereby become important
tools for your "inner physician."

Which route you take depends on your personal situation.
The main things is knowing that while you are wrestling with
this illness you can call upon many helpful and strong allies
waiting to be discovered and to be put to good use.

Erika Merz, MD, *is responsible for therapy advice at the Medical
Scientific Department of HELIXOR Heilmittel GmbH & Co. in
Rosenfeld, Germany. HELIXOR manufactures mistletoe preparations, sold in Europe. Physicians desiring information call the
therapy advisory service: 011 49 74 28 93 5-335 (fax 011 49 28
935-350 email: advice@helixor.de). This article was reprinted
courtesy of Helixor.*

Painting Therapy for Cancer Patients

Phoebe Alexander

IN ANTHROPOSOPHICAL MEDICINE, ILLNESSES can be viewed from the standpoint of the polarities of warm and cold—the loosening, dissolving, fever illnesses that predominate in childhood versus the hardening, sclerotic illnesses such as arthritis, heart disease, and cancer predominant in adulthood and old age.

Because humanity as a whole has now passed the midpoint of its development in terms of earthly evolution and is entering into its adulthood, even our children today are developing these cold illnesses. These are illnesses of our time rather than of personal karma, and there is only so much we can do to keep them at bay. Humanity no longer has the youthful vitality it once had in the days when the great fever plagues swept across continents. In the great chilling off process of aging and hardening, we are now much more vulnerable to auto-immune conditions such as Lupus, and diseases of weakened immunity, such as AIDS. But through the same processes, we have also evolved into more defined and unique individuals with active cognitive faculties. How do we recover this lost warmth to find healing for the future?

Mistletoe and the Tree

From out of his spiritual research, Rudolf Steiner pointed to the white-berried mistletoe, *Viscum album*, as the basis for the treatment of cancer. The plant, which grows on apple, oak, poplar, elm, pine, and fir trees, is now known to be a hemi- or holo-parasite living in symbiosis with its host tree (a true parasite weakens its host, eventually killing it, by sapping its vitality). These mistletoe-receptive trees tend to grow above or near to moving water, and rather than having caused the weakness of the tree, the mistletoe has been found to play a significant role in maintaining the life of the tree.

When mistletoe plants, thought to have been culprits in the trees' demise, were removed from their living but ailing hosts, the trees promptly died—often with split or burst limbs. The mistletoe was found to have functioned as kind of release valve for the pressure of superabundant growth forces that the tree alone could not contain or withstand. To put this in anthroposophical terms, the mistletoe receives its life from an overactivity or superfluity of etheric forces from the tree. So the mistletoe needs the tree, but the tree also needs the mistletoe.

Mistletoe and Mercury

According to Leen Mees, MD, of the Netherlands, Rudolf Steiner spoke of the mistletoe as a carry-over from Atlantean times when there were a greater number of in-between life forms—animal-plants and plant-animals—than are commonly found now on earth. Not having roots of its own, and being ball-formed—neither heliotropic nor geotropic—are two such characteristics. This ball-like form of the mistletoe further creates a sort of enclosed soul-space or astrality, common to the animal world. (The tumor also has such a form.) Further, the rhythmical pattern of its growth (contraction, the seed (●); expansion, the leaves (ᐱᐱ); contraction, the bud; expansion, the berry) are the qualities attributed to mercury in its tendencies to dispersion (expansion, or centrifugal activity) into multiple tiny droplets, and vapor, and its polar tendency toward pulling together (contraction, or centripetal activity) into a tight spherical form. Also, because mercury is the only metal which is liquid at room temperature, it is said to possess inner heat.

Color, Warmth and the Soul

Warmth is an astral or soul quality that we share with the animal world, especially with warm-blooded species, whose moods and whose tenderness toward their young strike a reflective note in our own souls. The astral body gives us our consciousness—our life of soul—our inner life, inner light, inner warmth. The warmth of the soul lives in feelings and moods—in the world of color. And it is only in the light of consciousness that color can be perceived.

Color is the language of the soul, and it finds its reflection in the colored world of outer nature. We find we are warmed within by the fiery glow of the setting sun even on a chilly evening, and will shiver a bit and reach for a sweater in the gathering blue dusk of evening, though the temperature may be quite warm. Our experience of inner temperature, or of soul mood, is strongly affected by the moods of outer nature, including the moods of those around us, and is experienced by the soul in color qualities, each with its own inner soul gesture.

The outward shining of yellow (⚘) (the color closest to light) and the inward shining of blue (⚘) (the color closest to darkness) are at the two poles of the expansion and contraction in the life of the soul. Mediating between the expansiveness of light (yellow) and the contracting darkness (blue), is warmth (red)—the warmth of our feeling life, the fire of our vitality and enthusiasm, the love of the heart.

Unlike light and darkness which remain in dynamic tension with one another, warmth can penetrate and permeate both light and darkness. Red, which is the color of warmth and activity, has its own inner contraction and expansion, its own inner mercurial activity like the beating or pulsating of the heart. It is in red, in this warmth element in the blood, that our human ego, our spirit, comes to dwell. This ego-imbued warmth gives us life and vitality, strengthens our etheric body, brings purpose and compassion to our soul, and enlivens our body. Light disperses darkness, and darkness can encroach upon light. Only our warmth can infuse them both.

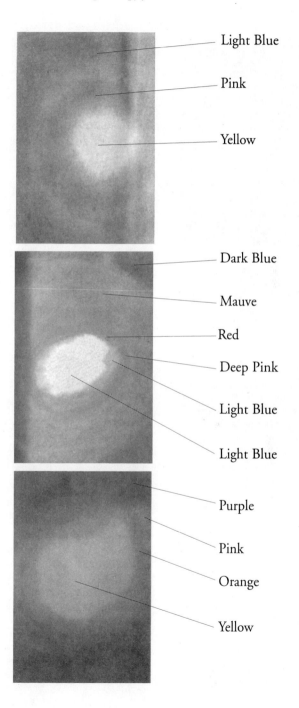

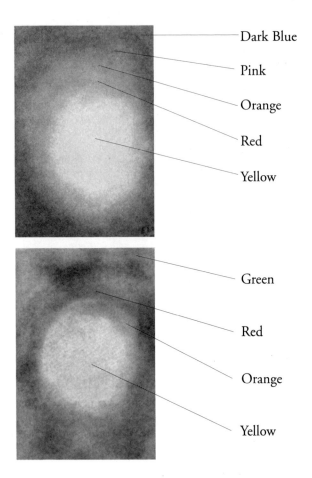

Dark Blue

Pink

Orange

Red

Yellow

Green

Red

Orange

Yellow

Painting Therapy and Iscador

Through conscious, intentional activity in thought and deed warmed by the forces of the heart, true healing can take place. From the mistletoe plant imagination, Iscador therapy has been developed from the plant substance itself for various cancers and for AIDS and likewise from the mistletoe imagination illustrated here was developed. While watercolor painting with prismatic colors has a general warming and dissolving effect, the particular painting exercise shown here (see opposite) requires that the individual make an effort of the will—powerful and difficult—first to find a balance between the light and the darkness (expressed by color intensity, and dimension and proportion of light and darkness), and then to bring a halo of warmth between the light and darkness, letting it first penetrate inward toward the source of the light, and then outward toward the coldest reaches of the darkness—warming the light and warming the darkness. Each time the exercise is repeated, an effort is made to spread the warmth a little further than the time before into whichever area it is having difficulty penetrating.

It is very visible from the illustrations that some individuals can bring their warmth into the light with ease, but not into the darkness, and vice versa. The aim is a balance of light and darkness, a palpable rather than a pale use of color, and a good penetration of the ego/warmth into both the light and darkness with an overall sense of harmoniousness and a breathing of the colors. Warmed light appears as orange or golden yellow—the saffron color of monks' robes—the color of spiritual joy. Warmed darkness appears as violet or purple—the color of the robes of kings—the color of spiritual wisdom. In this circular rainbow around our inner light, the green of the plant world (the etheric) is called up—activated—as an afterimage in our souls when we breathe in the spiritual love of red.

This exercise is always enormously gratifying as well as very meditative and inwardly activating. One is literally warmed by it. I use it frequently in my therapeutic painting group at The Fellowship Community in Spring Valley, NY as a general tonic, especially during the dark and cold winter months. When the basic exercise is completed, we may choose to make the source of light and warmth a candle flame, painting the candle downward from the flame to a table or bench below (blue)—a Christmas/Chanukah experience. At the beginning of February (Candlemas), we celebrate the pregnant earth by creating a cozy and warm hollow from which new life is preparing to emerge. Variations and manifestations of the theme are limited, or given flight, by the imagination.

Phoebe Alexander *studied Waldorf education at Emerson College in England and art therapy at "De Wervel" Academie voor Kunstinninge Therapie in Holland. She has a master's degree in therapeutic recreation and is a certified Recreational Therapist. Phoebe heads the Association for Anthroposophical Art Therapy.*

Life In the Balance

Louise Frazier

WHEN WE CONSIDER THE HUMAN ORGAN-
ism as constantly in a state of seeking balance—
that even in the development of cancer, a balance
is being sought in relation to internal or external forces—how
can nutrition best be applied? Nutrition is in the front line of
prevention, as many studies show today. In a recent series of
interviews with well-known personalities who overcame cancer,
a strict vegan plant-based diet was reportedly being followed
successfully in maintaining health. Nevertheless, in the very delicate process of achieving health-giving balance, glib answers
may be felt as insufficient. While a vegetarian diet based on
whole grains, fresh vegetables, and fruits indeed can be seen as
primary for optimal health and healing, how may we find the
more subtle threads to weave or reweave the warp and woof of

our physical garment for wellness? What approaches can be taken to ennoble our organism, our soul and spirit, even in the face of the darkness of life-threatening occurrences?

To begin with we can weave a measure of harmony into our sheaths by making foods of our local region in all its seasons the mainstay of our menu. This has the effect of connecting us with the in-breathing and out-breathing of the Earth where we live and breathe. Considering that pollution creates a toxic environment, eating food grown closer to home instead of trucked from far and wide, also makes sense.

Most important to protect us from the many manipulations by the food industry with all their unknown effects, is to choose biodynamic/organic foods. Throughout the country there is a growing movement towards foods grown in this manner, especially in CSA farms* and the small local farms whose produce fills Farmers' Markets in numerous towns. Streaming towards our metabolic system come dynamic forces or dullness accorded by the food we consume. The fabric of our whole being is thus colored and strengthened or left weakened and drab.

King Zarathustra, who guided ancient human beings into cultivation of the land, knew that cosmic forces in the Sun rayed into grains growing in the fields. He saw this effect radiating into the human being who ate grain, leading people to pause and reverently imagine: "The Sun will rise in you when you enjoy the fruits of the field." Think of what healing such imagination and reverence can bring to us in our daily meals! There is no doubt that these first fruits of cultivation—the seven grains—have brought powerful nourishment to humankind from earliest times. That nourishment is still available to us today through organic agricultural practices. Steaming dishes of rice, sunny millet, barley and oats are foods to nurture the hale and hearty, as well as the frail and ill—young or old can experience enveloping warmth, balance, and strength in simple whole grain foods.

Emaciated refugees, and later whole orphanages of children, were restored to health through the work of German medical doctor nutritionist, Werner Kollath. He fed them a diet based on fresh grains, especially wheat berries cracked in a heavy old coffee grinder, which those finding health again referred to as "Dr. Kollath's miracle machine." Soaking the grains in water for five to ten hours and adding a grated apple or other fruit, raisins, nuts, and honey was the miracle food. Research showed his fresh-grain "muesli" to have regenerative qualities.

A similar breakfast can simply be made by soaking overnight a third of a cup of organic steel cut oats in a bowl with half a cup of fresh cold water topped with a saucer and set aside on the counter at room temperature. In the morning add grated or chopped fresh fruits or whole berries of the season–or soaked dried organic fruits such as apples, apricots, pears, along with one tablespoon each of sunflower seeds or chopped nuts, raisins, fresh lemon juice, and one teaspoon of honey, if desired. All the better if one has a grain mill and can grind the grains fresh each time. After ten hours in water, fermentation sets in and then the grains must be cooked or discarded, but even when cooked, good nourishment can be found. For frail elders, such a cooked porridge is ideal, especially with honey added to uplift the will to life and bring comfort.

Oats help connect the spirit to the physical, enabling us to go beyond the materialist world that confronts us everywhere. Dishes of millet are noteworthy as well—not only are they easily assimilable, but they have grounding qualities that bring us down to earth so we can meet the challenges of our lives. We might also find enlightenment with barley included in our weekly menu, as it has been found to keep us awake in our head, both by the Greeks and in today's research. Rounding out the preferred foods of a diet for cancer prevention and healing are lactic acid-fermented vegetables—sauerkraut being familiar to most of us. Red beets cultured in this manner especially have shown to be healing in work with cancer. Doctors in Europe have found a lessening of cancer cells, shrinking and even disappearance of tumors in patients who consumed lactic acid cultured beets each day. In addition a resurgence of vitality is often experienced as well.

Following the clock can be advantageous, clothing us in rhythm, through eating our three or five small daily meals at the same time. The liver thrives on regular rhythms and the whole metabolism will benefit thereby. To wrap up, it is highly recommended that we eat between seven am and seven pm, allowing twelve hours of fasting overnight. This will enable our organism to fully digest our foods and cleanse us from toxins. Then as we sleep at night, our soul will more readily knit up our physical body in its restorative task, while our spirit is making its trip out into the starry world where the welcoming cosmos carries out activities to help us develop and meet the new day. Thus we might better create a fitting fabric for healing in our life, instead of haphazardly hanging by a thread.

Louise Frazier *is a nutritionist and lecturer in Albany, New York. This article is reprinted with permission from LILIPOH #16.*

*Community Supported Agriculture, where a share in the harvest can be purchased. Call the Bio-Dynamic Association of America (1-800-516-7797) for the address of one in your area or to order biodynamic foods by mail.

Resources

A Daily Menu
Suggestions Aimed at Cancer Prevention

Breakfast

1. Muesli made from grain flakes with honey, nuts, apples (fruit in season), and soured milk.
2. Porridge with the same ingredients.
3. Freshly ground grains soaked overnight, cooked in the same water, and left to absorb the moisture. Add same ingredients.
4. Wholegrain bread, butter with quark* or cheese or (if sweetness is craved) fruit concentrates or honey. An apple or fruit in season. Beverage: herb tea.

Lunch

1. Cup of vegetable broth, or bitter tea, or warmed lactic-fermented vegetable juice.
2. Raw vegetables or salad.
3. Grain dishes, alternating each day. Cooked or raw vegetables cooked or raw to go with the grains. Sauce made with herb. If desired and suitable, various milk puddings, a quark* dessert or stewed fruit.

Evening Meals

1. Soup made with freshly ground grains and either herbs or stewed dried fruits.
2. Soured milk products such as buttermilk or kefir.
3. Bread, butter, light cheeses, herb tea.

Between meals: herb teas, crisp bread, wholemeal biscuits, fruit, nuts, honey, fruit juices, soured milk products, lactic fermented vegetable juice.

From: Diet and Cancer *by Udo Renzenbrink (The Anthroposophic Press, $11.95 paperback).*

quark: a soured milk product (fromage frais). You can easily make it at home by suspending yogurt in a muslin bag until the whey has run out.

* * *

A New Study of Iscador

Mistletoe Therapy found to be Effective in Cancer (see reference #32)

A major thirty-year-long study with more than 35,000 participants reports that extract of mistletoe (Iscador) greatly improves survival rate for a wide variety of cancers, including breast cancer. Study participants who augmented conventional therapy with mistletoe extract survived forty percent longer compared with those who didn't use the plant therapy.

"This is a far-reaching, landmark study with significant results," says David Riley, M.D., Editor in Chief of *Alternative Therapies in Health and Medicine*, the leading peer-reviewed journal on complementary and alternative medicine, which published the study in its May 2001 issue.

The study, "Viscum Album in Cancer Treatment: A Systematic Epidemiology Investigation," followed 35,000 residents of Heidelberg, Germany over thirty years, identifying five thousand who had cancer. Then the researchers matched more than 300 pairs of participants who had a similar type and stage of disease. One group took mistletoe extract in addition to conventional treatment; the other group took conventional treatment alone. After comparing the length of survival, the study concludes that participants who added mistletoe extract to their treatment lived forty percent longer than those who did not.

Alternative Therapies in Health and Medicine, the leading peer-reviewed journal on complementary and alternative medicine, is also publishing abstracts of ten other recent studies on the effectiveness of mistletoe extract for cancer.

Alternative Therapies will make study authors and other experts available for interviews. Contact: Sheldon Lewis, Inner Doorway, 646-336-1919

We thank David Riley, MD for the following references:

Mistletoe has been reviewed by experts at the National Institutes of Health as an adjunctive complementary treatment for cancer.

1. A review of mistletoe use in cancer was completed by the University of Texas Center for Alternative Medicine Research in Cancer in 1997 by Mary Ann Richardson, PhD. Currently she is a program officer at the NIH— National Center for Complementary and Alternative Medicine in Bethesda, Maryland.

2. Dr. Jeffery White, Director of the Office of Cancer Complementary and Alternative Medicine at the National Cancer Institute, in 1998 provided an overview of mistletoe to the Cancer Advisory Panel (CAP) of the NIH Office of Alternative Medicine. Dr. White noted that the scientific literature suggests that mistletoe may have anti-tumor effects and may enhance survival.

* * *

Natural Products During Recovery

Weleda

When life forces are depleted and the organism is struggling with illness we need the support of a nurturing environment and natural lifestyle.

In Weleda products, fragrant essential oils have been combined with beneficial natural substances to enliven both soul and body. Whether in a clinic or at home, you will feel your spirits lifted and find renewed energy with Weleda oils or creams.

Rosemary's invigorating aroma in shampoo and soap will help you take hold of your body in the morning. If you have difficulty falling asleep, Lavender Bath Oil or Milk will help you relax, and create the right transition for night. If your legs or feet feel swollen and tired, try Citrus Leg Toner or Foot Cream, with refreshing citrus aromatic oils and toning witch hazel.

Our skin mirrors what is taking place in the soul (fright causes pallor, anger causes redness) and also mirrors the substances we absorb. Conventional cancer therapy depletes skin moisture so that it loses its elasticity. Nourishing creams and soothing ointments are even more necessary than usual to counter balance these damaging effects.

Weleda's Iris Face Care Line helps harmonize and protect skin moisture. For those with very sensitive skin the fragrance-free Almond Face Care Line with sweet almond oil is particularly suited. In cases of radiation treatment, Burn Care, a soothing and cooling homeopathic ointment in a natural vegetable base, will help relieve the burning sensation.

For further information call Weleda at (800) 241-1030.

—*Michele Sanz-Cardona*

Dr. Hauschka

Dr. Hauschka Skin Care offers a variety of preparations that are particularly comforting during times of healing and recovery from cancer. The restoration of personal well being is achieved through the use of products that offer warming, protecting and renewing qualities. Products that encourage warmth and are beneficial for symptoms of exhaustion and deficient circulation include Sage Bath and Rosemary Leg and Arm Toner. Sage Bath is most effective when used as a footbath four times per week. The foot treatment should last seven to twenty minutes while increasing the temperature of the bath over the course of the week to 105 degrees Fahrenheit. Rosemary Leg and Arm Toner may be applied daily to the feet, legs, and arms for lasting comfort.

The qualities of the rose, long known for its ability to harmonize and protect, are amplified in Rose Day Cream and Rose Body Moisturizer. Rose Day Cream is most effective for daily facial protection. It relieves the symptoms of sensitive, reddened, dry and flaking skin, leaving a velvety-soft and tender feeling much appreciated during recovery. The luxurious composition of ingredients in Rose Body Moisturizer provides a protective sheath with a warming and harmonizing effect for those in stressful situations or for when the nerves are overtaxed. The Moor Lavender Body Oil offers additional protection while the patient renews vitality.

Dr. Hauschka's Rhythmic Night Conditioner encourages healthy skin renewal and is beneficial for symptoms of connective tissue weakness and wrinkle formation during extended illness. Apply to the face and neck nightly after cleansing for a period of twenty-eight days or until the condition improves.

For further information call Dr. Hauschka at (800) 247-9907.—*Susan Kurz*

* * *

Anthroposophical Resources for Iscador

Weleda
USA distributors of Iscador (Iscar) has manufactured anthroposophical medicines and body care products since 1921. It is a member of the American Association of Homeopathic Pharmacists and its principals been associated with the Homeopathic Pharmacopea Convention of the United States since 1974. For inquiries call (800) 241-1030 or write Weleda Inc., 175 Route 9W North, Congers, NY 10920. www.weleda.com

Hiscia, Society for Cancer Research
A not for profit organization manufactures Iscador. For a complete list of research papers and other information on Iscador write: Hiscia, 4144 Arlesheim, Switzerland or call: 011-41-61-701-2324. www.hiscia.ch

Physicians Association for Anthroposophical Medicine (PAAM)
1923 Geddes Avenue
Ann Arbor, MI 48104-1797
Phone: (734) 930-9462, Fax: (734) 662-1727
Email: paam@anthroposophy.org

* * *

A Partial List of Representative Physicians Working with Iscador

Northeast
Tom Cowan, MD, 69 Main Street, Peterborough, NH 03458
(603) 924-3644

Anna Lups, MD, Pleroma Farms, Clinic and Retreat
Box 149, Route 14, Hudson, NY 12534
(518) 828-3292

Gerald Karnow, MD and Kent Hesse, MD
Fellowship Community Associates
241 Hungry Hollow Road, Spring Valley, NY 10977
(914) 366-8494

Ira Cantor, MD, Center for Integrative Medicine
3900 Ford Road, Philadelphia PA 19131
(215) 879-5121

Richard Fried, MD, Kimberton Clinic
800 Hare's Hill Road, Kimberton, PA 19442
(610) 933-0708

South
Mark J. Eisen, MD, Airport Road, Suite A,
Chapel Hill, NC 27514
(919) 967-9452

Andrea Pautz, MD, Jacksonville, Florida.
(904) 246-3583
Robert Zieve, MD, Fox Hollow Clinic
8909 Highway 329, Crestwood, KY 40014
(502) 241-4304

Midwest
Quentin McMullen, MD and Molly McMullen-Laird, MD
Community Supported Anthroposophical Medicine and
Patient Summer Retreat
23855 S. Huron Parkway, Ann Arbor, MI 48104
(734) 677-7990

Ross Rentea, MD and Andrea Rentea, MD
Paulina Medical Clinic
3525 W. Petersen, Chicago, IL 60659
(773) 583-7793

Rocky Mountains
Philip Incao, MD, Steiner Medical Center
1624 Gilpin Street, Denver, CO 80218-1633
(303) 321-2100

West Coast
Bruno Seemann, MD
1334 West Valley Parkway, Escondido, CA 92029
(760) 740-0707

Raphael House
7953 California Avenue, Fair Oaks, CA 95628
(916) 967-8250

* * *

Contacts for Anthroposophical Therapists

These therapies should only be practiced in conjunction with a licensed medical professional.

The Anthroposophical Nurses Association of America (ANAA)

Anthroposophical nursing extends the traditional art and science of nursing to reflect a more complete picture of the developing human being. Anthroposophical nurses recognize the human being as a spiritual being in a human body. They walk with patients on their unique journey toward healing and know that the healing process ultimately rests within each individual. A course of study for registered nurses is available. 1923

Geddes Avenue, Ann Arbor, MI 48104, (734) 994-8303.
ANAANurses@aol.com

Artemisia

The Association for the Anthroposophical Renewal of
Healing
1923 Geddes Avenue, Ann Arbor, MI 48104, (734) 761-
5172. artemisia@anthroposophy.org
A resource of all anthroposophical therapists in the US. Call
for information.

Association for Therapeutic Eurythmy in North America (ATHENA)

Eurythmy is an art of movement that brings the inner dynamics of speech and music to expression through movement and
gesture. Its branch, therapeutic eurythmy, is an essential component of anthroposophically extended medicine. It allows the
individual to actively participate in the prevention and treatment of illness. Therapeutic eurythmy is an uplifting and
inspiring patient resource. Ann Cook, 1081 Dickens Drive,
Santa Rose, CA 95401, (707) 568-4288.

Creative Speech

Creative Speech is an artistic practice, working with the vitality
and healing forces of the spoken word. The inherent gesture
and movement in speech are engaged through the rhythms and
styles of poetry and prose. These tools strengthen and free both
breath and voice, providing a basis for numerous health-giving
benefits. Contact: The Speech Association of North America:
Judith Pownall, (312) 565-2477.

Dorion School of Music Therapy
The task of music as healer is to rekindle the memory of the
tonal world from which we all were formed. In learning to listen
actively and to create sounds, the patient is led into his/her own
deeper beingness. For this the lyre, a string instrument, is ideally
suited. With simple exercises the music therapist creates a
healing atmosphere, gradually fulfilling the silent longing to be
in harmony with one's body and with the world. 1784 Fairview
Road, Glenmoore, PA 19343

**Federation of Natural Medicine Users in North America
(Fonmuna)**
PO Box 237, Congers, NY 10920, (845) 268-2627
www.fonmuna.org

Movement Therapy
An anthroposophically oriented movement therapy and discipline
applied by several hundred practitioners worldwide and recognized by the International Somatic Movement Education and
Therapy Association (ISMETA). Spatial Dynamics plays a supportive role for those receiving medical treatment for cancer and
related disorders, concentrating on post-operative movement
therapy and helping to get patients back on their feet and moving
with greater ease. Spatial Dynamics Institute, Inc., 129 Hayes
Road, Grangerville, NY 12871, (518) 325-7096
Email: spadyninst@aol.com, www.spacialdynamics.com

School for Rhythmical Massage
Understanding that rhythm brings healing, this massage was

developed in the 1920s by Dr. Ita Wegman, who refined elaborate qualities of touch, enhancing the forces of lightness and levity through lifting and suction. At times when the pressures of life and illness weigh people down, the rhythmic, delicate quality of this form of treatment is a great help. School for Rhythmical Massage, PO Box 825, Kimberton, PA 19442 (610) 469-9689

Therapeutic Association for Anthroposophical Art Therapy in North America. (AAATA)
Goethe describes color as movement and activity arising where light and darkness meet. Light and darkness are reflections of the human being—the light of the ego meeting the darkness of substance. In diagnostic drawing and painting, done in a supportive setting, light, darkness, and color becomes outer representations revealing inner movement. It can become an important part of healing. 138 West 15th Street, New York, NY 10011, (212) 744-0247. artopathy@aol.com
www.phoenixartsgroup.org/aaatna/index.html

* * *

Anthroposophical Hospitals and Clinics

Germany
Filder Klinik im Haberschlai 7
70794 Filderstadt
T: 011 49 711 7703 0
F: 011 49 711 7703 3679

Friedrich-Husemann Klinik
Psychiatrisch-Neurologische Klinik
79256 Buchenbach
T: 011 49 7661 3920
F: 011 49 7661 39414

Gemeinschaftskrankenhaus
Gerhard-Kienle-Weg Herdecke
5831 3 Herdecke/Ruhr
T: 011 49 2330 62 1
F: 011 49 2330 62 3995

Gemeinschaftskrankenhaus
Kladower Damm 221
14089 Berlin Havelshoehe
T: 011 49 30 36501 0
F: 011 49 30 36501 444

Klinik Oeschelbronn
Am Eichhof 75223
Niefern-Oeschelbronn
T: 011 49 7233 68 0
F: 011 49 7233 68 110

Paracelsus-Krankenhaus
Burghaldenweg 60
75378 Bad Liebenzell/Unterl.
T: 011 49 7052 925 0
F: 011 49 7052 925 215

Hospitals with Anthroposophical Wards in Germany
Knappschafts-Krankenhaus
Am Deimelsberg 34a
45276 Essen
Essen-Steele
T: 011 49 201 80546 01
F: 011 49 201 80546 03

Krankenhaus Lahnhoehe
Am Kurpark 1
56112 Lahnstein
T: 011 49 2621 91 5 0
F: 011 49 2621 91 5 575

Krankenhaus Rissen
Suurheid 20
22559 Hamburg
T: 011 49 40 8191
F: 011 49 40 8130 19

Kreiskrankenhaus Heidenhaim
Schlosshaussstrasse 100
89522 Heidenheim
T: 011 49 7321 332 502
F: 011 49 7321 332 048

Switzerland
Lukas Klinik
Brachmattstrasse 19
Onkologische Spezial-Klinik
CH-4144 Arlesheim
T: 011 41 61 706 7171
F: 011 41 61 706 7173

Ita Wegman-Klinik
Pfeffinger Weg 1
CH-4144 Arlesheim
T: 011 41 61 705 7111
F: 011 41 61 705 0274

Paracelsus-Spital
Bergstrasse 16
CH-8805 Richterswil
T: 011 41 1 787 2121
F: 011 41 1 787 2351

* * *

Books & Videos

From Mercury Press

Mercury Press is associated with the Fellowship Community. It carries an extensive list of books on the anthroposophical approach to health and illness, of which three books are listed below. For a complete catalog, write to: Mercury Press, 241 Hungry Hollow Road, Spring Valley, NY 10977, or call (845) 425-9357.

Anthroposophical Medicine and Therapies for Cancer
edited by Hans Richard Heiligtag, MD. 85 pages, $7.95 paperback.

With contributions by physicians, researchers, nutritionists and nurses, and art therapists. Topics include the rationale for mistletoe therapy including the results of research, physical therapy, biographical work, and the seven arts as aids to healing.

An Anthroposophical Approach to Cancer: Six Lectures by
Rita Leroi, MD. 45 pages, $5.50 paperback.

The broadest possible view of cancer is one which includes spiritual questions of destiny relative to individual and social evolution. In this advanced anthroposophical material, Dr. Leroi covers cancer as an aid of destiny, the treatment of the cancer patient, mistletoe treatments of cancer, and the Lukas Clinic in Arlesheim, Switzerland.

Cancer: A Mandate to Humanity by Friedrich Lorenz, MD. 39 pages, $5.50 paperback.

Here is a view of cancer that focuses not on the illness, but on the human being who is going through the experience. It discusses cancer as a disease of our time and highlights the limitations of the popular "cellular view" of the sickness as a "catastrophe of form."

Diet and Cancer by U. Renzenbrink. 71 pages, $7.95 paperback.

Describes aspects of metabolism, the function of the liver, the specific qualities of different basic foods and their use, tried and proven diets, and much more.

From Fonmuna

Fonmuna (Federation of Natural Medicine Users in North America) provides the following books. Write Fonmuna, PO Box 237, Congers, NY 10920 or call (845) 268-2627. www.fonmuna.org

Iscador by Robert W. Gorter, MD. 82 pages, $12.00 paperback.

Includes mistletoe development, toxic substances, research, clinical research, uses and aims of mistletoe treatment, and different applications. Ideal as a table reference and guide for physicians and introductory orientation for patients.

Lukas Clinic Cookery Book. 71 pages, $7.95 paperback. Compiled by the Society for Cancer Research. This small book contains a large variety of tasty and wholesome meals.

A Slice of Life by Lee Sturgeon-Day. 147 pages. $10.95 paperback. An inspirational, personal story of healing through cancer with Iscador.

Treatment with Iscador: The First Steps (video). A Wolfgang Jung Video, Verlag für GanzheitsMedizin, 26 mins. $26.00.
This video shows the practical help mistletoe can offer a patient after an operation, chemotherapy, or radiotherapy. It provides important basic information on mistletoe therapy and shows what the patient can do to actively further the healing process.

From the Mistletoe Plant to the Anti-Cancer Medication: Iscador. A Wolfgang Jung Video, Verlag für GanzheitsMedizin, 25 mins. $26.00.
This film focuses on the botanical features of the mistletoe and its strange seasonal growth pattern, its cultivation on host trees, some of which are very rare, and its processing (also with regard to the anti-tumor substances it contains).

For Medical Doctors

Iscador: Investigator's Brochure. *Viscum Album* Research in Progress. Revised January 1999.

Annual Report of the Society for Cancer Research: 1980, 1981, 1982, 1983. (May be ordered from Verein für Krebforschung. CH-4144, Arlesheim).

From Lantern Books

Practical Home Care Medicine: A Natural Approach edited by Christine Murphy. 96 pages, $10.00 paperback.

This book is a special resource guide compiled from the notes and experiences of natural healers and physicians, listing some of their most frequently used home care medicines, herbal teas, and kitchen remedies. Other sections include: the healing environment, first aid hints, fever, medical supplies for the home kit, the basic medicine kit, foot baths, and other important resources.

A Race for Life: A Diet and Exercise Program for Superfitness and Reversing the Aging Process by Ruth E. Heidrich, Ph.D. 192 pages. $15.95 paperback.

In her mid-forties, Ruth Heidrich was diagnosed with breast cancer. After undergoing a double mastectomy, she challenged herself to the punishing Ironman Triathlon, a test of endurance involving a 2.4-mile swim, 112-mile bike ride, and a 26.2-mile marathon run. Twenty years later, Heidrich is still running, cancer-free, and positive about life. This is her story. She describes her fight with cancer, the healing powers of proper nutrition, and the rewards of running the toughest races in the world.

* * *

Mistletoe References for Physicians

1. Addington-Hall J.M., MacDonald L.D., Anderson H.R.: "Can the Spitzer Quality of Life Index help to reduce prognostic uncertainty in terminal care?" **Br J Cancer** Oct, 62(4):695–9, 1990.

2. Awwad S., Cull A., Gregor A.: "Long-term survival in adult hemispheric glioma: prognostic factors and quality of outcome." **Clin Oncol (R Coll Radiol)** Nov 2(6):343–6, 1990.

3. Bauman G.S., Gaspar L.E., Fisher B.J., Halperin E.C., Macdonald D.R., Cairncross J.G.: "A prospective study of short-course radiotherapy in poor prognosis glioblastoma multiforme." **Int J Radiat Oncol Biol Phys** 29:835–839, 1994.

4. Beuth J., Ko H.L., Gabius H.J., Burrichter H., Oette K., Pulverer G. "Behavior of lymphocyte subsets and expression of activation markers in response to immunotherapy with galactoside specific lectin from mistletoe in breast cancer patients." **Clin Investig** 70:658–61, 1992.

5. Beuth J., Ko H.L., Gabius H.J., Pulverer G. "Influence of treatment with the immunomodulatory effective dose of the b-galactoside specific lectin from mistletoe on tumor colonization in BALB/c-mice for two experimental model systems." **In Vivo** 5(1):29–32, 1991.

6. Beyersdorff D., Irmey G. "Die kostenerstattung biologischer heilmittel bei krebserkrankungen in der arztlichen praxis." **Erfahrungsheilkunde** 82–90, 1996.

7. Böhringer B. Personal communication to principal investigator. March 29, 2001.

8. Boie 1980.

9. Boie D., Gutsch J. "Helixor in cancer of colon and rectum." **Schriftenreihe Krebsgeschehen** 23:65–76, 1980.

10. Bruera E., Neumann C.M. "Management of specific symptom complexes in patients receiving palliative care." **CMAJ** 158(13):1717–26, 1998.

11. Buhl K., Schlag P., Herfarth, C. "Quality of life and functional results following different types of resection for gastric carcinoma." **Eur J Surg Oncol** 16:404–409, 1990.

12. Burger A.M., Mengs U., Schüler J.B., Zinke H., Lentzen H. and Fiebig H.H. "Recombinant mistletoe lectin (ML) is a potent inhibitor of tumor cell growth in vitro and in vivo." **Proceedings of the American Association for Cancer Research** 40:399–399, 1999.

13. Büssing A. *Mistletoe. The Genus Viscum.* Amsterdam: Harwood Academic Publishers, 2001.

14. Büssing A. Azhari A., Ostendorp H., Lehnert A., Schweizer K. "*Viscum album* L. estracts reduce sister chromatid exchanges in cultured peripheral blood mononuclear cells." **Eur J Cancer** 30A:1836–1841, 1994.

15. Büssing A., Regnery A., Schweizer K. "Effects of *Viscum album* L. on cyclophosphamide-treated peripheral blood mononuclear cells *in vitro*: Sister chromatid exchanges and activation/proliferation marker expression." **Cancer Letters**. 94:199–205, 1995.

16. Bussing A., Suzart K., Bergmann J., Pfuller U., Schietzel M., Schweizer K. "Induction of apoptosis in human lym-

phocytes treated with *Viscum album* L. is mediated by the mistletoe lectins." **Cancer Letters** 99:59–72, 1996.

17. Bussing A. "Mistletoe: a story with an open end." **Anti-Cancer Drugs (Suppl)** 8:S1-S2, 1997.

18. Clark W.C.: "Pain sensitivity and the report of pain." **Anesthesiology** 40:272–275, 1977.

19. Cleeland C.S.: "Measurement and prevalence of pain in cancer." **Semin Oncol Nurs** 1:87–96, 1985.

20. Daut R., Cleeland C., Flanery R. "Development of the Wisconsin Brief Pain questionnaire to assess pain in cancer and other diseases." **Pain** 17:197–210, 1983.

21. Dold U., et al. "Krebszusatztherapie beim fortgeschrittenen nicht-kleinzelligen Bronchialkarzinom," Stuttgart-New York: Georg Thieme Verlag. 1991, pp. 1–144.

22. Endo Y., Tsuguri K., Franz H.: "The site of action of the A chain of mistletoe lectin on eukaryotic ribosomes." **FEBS Letters** 231(2): 378–380, 1988.

23. Elsasser-Beile U.; Voss M.; Schuhle R.; Wetterauer U. "Biological effects of natural and recombinant mistletoe lectin and an aqueous mistletoe extract on human monocytes and lymphocytes in vitro." **J Clin Lab Anal** 14(6):255–9, 2000.

24. Ferrell B.R., Rhiner M., Cohen, M., Grant, M. "Pain as a metaphor for illness. Part I: impact of cancer pain on family caregivers." **Onc Nurs Forum** 18 (8);1303–1309, 1991.

25. Franz H., Friemel H., Buchwald S., Palntikow A., Kopp J., Korner I.J. "The A chain of lectin I from European mistletoe (*Viscum album*) induces interleukin-I and interleukin-II in human mononuclear cells." **Lectins Biol Biochem**

7:247–250, eds. Kocourek J., Freed D.L.J. St. Louis, MO: Sigma Chemical Company, 1990.

26. Friess H., Beger H.G., Kunz N., Schilling M., Buchler M.W. "Treatment of advanced pancreatic cancer with mistletoe: results of a pilot trial." **Anticancer Res** 16(2):915–20, 1996.

27. Gabius H.J., et al. "The risk potential of alternative (herbal) medicine: tumor stimulation by mistletoe lectin present in proprietary extracts." Abstract #1151. **Proceedings of the American Association for Cancer Research**, 2001.

28. Glaus A. "Assessment of fatigue in cancer and non-cancer patients and in healthy individuals." **Support Care Cancer** 1:305–315, 1993.

29. Gorter R.W., van Wely M., Reif M., Stoss M. "Tolerability of an extract of European mistletoe among immuno-compromised and healthy individuals." **Alt Ther Health Med** 5:37–48, 1999.

30. Gray A.M.; Flatt P.R. "Insulin-secreting activity of the traditional antidiabetic plant *Viscum album* (mistletoe)." **J Endocrinol** Mar 160(3):409–14, 1999.

31. Grossarth-Maticek R., Kiene H., Baumgartner S.M., Vetter H. "*Viscum album* (Iscador) in cancer treatment. A systemic epidemiology investigation: Prospective Non-randomized and Randomized matched-pair studies nested within a cohort study." **Altern Ther Health Med**. 7:3, 2001.

32. Hajto T., Hostanka K., Fornalski M., Kirsch A. "Antitumorale aktivität des immunmodulatorisch wirkenden beta-galactosidspezifischen mistellektins bei der klin-

ischen anwendung von mistelextrakten (Iscador)." **Dtsch Z Onkologie** 23:1–6, 1991.

33. Hajto T., Hostanka K., Steinberg F., Gabius H.J.: "b-galactoside specific lectin from clinically applied mistletoe extract reduces tumor growth by augmentation of host defense system." **Blut** 61:164, 1990a.

34. Hajto T., Hostanska K., Frei K., Rordorf H.J., Gabius H.J.: "Increased secretion of tumor necrosis factor, interleukin 1, and interleukin 6 by human mononuclear cells exposed to b-galactoside-specific lectin from clinically applied mistletoe extract." **Cancer Res** 50:3322–6, 1990b.

35. Hajto T. "Immunomodulatory effects of Iscador: A *Viscum album* preparation." **Oncolog** 43(suppl 1):52–65, 1986.

36. Hajto T.; Hostanska K.; Saller. "Mistletoe therapy from the pharmacologic perspective." **Forsch Komplementarmed** Aug 6(4):186–94, 1999.

37. Hamprecht K., Handgretinger R., Voetsch W., Anderer F.A. "Mediation of human NK-activity by components in extracts of *Viscum album*." **Int.J.Immunopharmac** 9, 199–209, 1987.

38. Hauser S.P. "Mistel: Wunderkraut oder medikament? Klinische anwendung von mistlepräparaten in der onkologie." **Therapiewoche** 43:76–81, 1993a.

39. Hauser S.P. "Unproven methods in cancer treatment." **Curr Opinion Oncol** 5:646–54, 1993b.

40. Heiny B.M., Albrecht V. "Komplementäre Therapie mit Mistellektin-1-normiertem Extrakt. Lebensqualitätsstabilisierung beim fortgeschrittenen kolorektalen Karzinom—

Fakt oder Fiktion?" **Die Medizinische Welt** 48:419–423, 1997.

41. Heiny B.M., Beuth J. "Mistletoe extract standardized for the galactoside-specific lectin (ML-I) induces b-endorphin release and immunopotentiation in breast cancer patients." **Anticancer Res** 14:1339–1342, 1994.

42. Heiny B.M. "Additive Therapie mit standardisiertem Mistelextrakt reduziert die Leukopenie und verbessert die Lebensqualität von Patientinnen mit fortgeschrittenem Mammakarzinom unter palliativer Chemotherapie (VEC-Schema)." **Krebsmedizin** 12:1–14, 1991.

43. Hostanka K., Hajto T., Spagnoli G.C., Fischer J., Lentzen H., Herrmann R. "A plant lectin derived from *Viscum album* induces cytokine gene expression and protein production in cultures of human peripheral blood mononuclear cells." **Natural Immunity** 14:295–304, 1995.

44. Ingham, J.M., Foley, D.M. "Pain and the barriers to its relief at the end of life: a lesson for improving end of life health care." **Hosp J.** 89–100, 1998.

45. Jung M.L., Frantz M., Ribéreau-Gayon G., Anton R. "Die Mistellektine: Einfluss von Serum und Kohlenhydraten auf die Zytotoxizität und Stimuliering der Zytokin-produktion." In *Grundlagen der Misteltherapie. Aktueller Stand der Forschung und klinische Anwendung*, eds. R. Scheer, H. Becker and P.A. Berg) pp. 302–314, Edition Forschung (Karl und Veronica Carstens-Stiftung), Stuttgart: Hippokrates Verlag GmbH, 1996.

46. Jurin M., Zarkovic N., Borovic S., Kissel D. "Immunomodulation by the *Viscum album* L. preparation

Isorel and its antitumorous effects. In *Grundlagen der Misteltherapie. Aktueller Stand der Forschung und klinische Anwendung*, eds. R. Scheer, H. Becker and P.A. Berg) pp. 315–324, Edition Forschung (Karl und Veronica Carstens-Stiftung), Stuttgart: Hippokrates Verlag GmbH, 1996.

47. Jurin M., Zarkovic N., Hrzenjak M., Ilic Z. "Antitumorous and immunomodulatory effects of the *Viscum album* L. preparation Isorel." **Oncology** 50:393–398, 1993.

48. Kaegi E. "Unconventional therapies in cancer: 3. Iscador." **CMAJ** 158:1157–1159, 1998.

49. Khwaja T.A., Dias C.B., Pentecost S. "Recent studies on the anticancer activities of Mistletoe (*Viscum album*) and its alcaloids." **Oncology** 43, 42–50 (1986).

50. Kiene H. "Klinische Studien zur Misteltherapie karzinomatöser Erkankungen: Eine Übersicht." **Therapeutikon** 3(6):347–53, 1989.

51. Kleijnen J., Knipschild P. "Mistletoe treatment for cancer: Review of controlled trials in humans." **Phytomedicine** 1:255–260, 1994.

52. Klein-Franke A., Anderer F.A. "IL-12-mediated activation of MHC-unrestricted cytotoxicity of human PBMC subpopulations: Synergistic action of a plant rhamno-galacturonan." **Anticancer Research** 2511–2516, 1995.

53. Klett C.Y., Anderer F.A. "Activation of natural killer cell cytotoxicity of human blood monocytes by a low molecular weight component from viscum album extract." **Arzneim-Forsch/Drug Res** 39(II):1–20, 1989.

54. Koch F.E. "Experimentelle Untersuchungen über entzundungs und nekroseerzeugende Wirkung von *Viscum album*." **Z exp Med** 103:740–9, 1938.

55. Kovacs E., Hajto T., Hostanska K. "Improvement of DNA repair in lymphocytes of breast cancer patients treated with Viscum album extract (Iscador)." **Europ J Cancer** 27:1672–1676, 1991.

56. Kubasova T., Pfuller U., Koteles G.J., Csollak M., Eifler R. "Comparative studies on some cellular and immunological effects of mistletoe isolectin in vitro." In *Lectins: Biology, Biochemistry*, Vol 11, pp. 240–44. eds, Van Driessche E., Rouge P., Beeckmans S., Bog-Hansen T.C. Hellerup, Denmark:Textop, 1996.

57. Kuehn, J.J., Löhmer, H., Sommer, H., Fornalski, M., and Kindermann, G. "Prospectiv randomisierte Prüfung der Wirksamkeit und Verträglichkeit einer adjuvanten Misteltherapie (Iscador®) bei Nachbestrahlung nach Mammakarzinomoperation." 2000 (Contact Ischia).

58. Kunze E., Schulz H., Ahrens H., Gabius H.J. "Lack of an antitumoral effect of immunomodulatory galactoside-specific mistletoe lectin on N-methyl-N-nitrosourea-induced urinary bladder carcinogenesis in rats." **Exp.Toxic Pathol** 49:167–180, 1997.

59. Kunze E., Schulz H., and Gabius H.J. "Inability of galactoside-specific mistletoe lectin to inhibit N-methyl-N-nitrosourea-induced tumor development in the urinary bladder of rats and to mediate a local cellular immune response after long-term administration." **J. Cancer Res. Clin. Oncol.** 124:73–87, 1998.

60. Kuttan G., Kuttan R., "Immunological mechanism of action of the tumor reducing peptide from mistletoe extract (NSC 635089) cellular proliferation." **Cancer Letters** 123–130 (1992).

61. Kuttan G., Kuttan R. "Reduction of leukopenia in mice by Viscum album administration during radiation and chemotherapy." **Tumori** 79:74–76, 1993.

62. Kuttan G., Vasudevan D.M., Kuttan R. "Isolation and identification of a tumor reducing component from mistletoe extract." **Cancer Letters** 307–314, 1988.

63. Lange O., Scholz G., Gutsch J. "Modulation of the subjective and objective toxicity of aggressive radiochemotherapy with Helixor." Unpublished Study.

64. Lenartz D., Stoffel B., Menzel J., Beuth J. "Immunoprotective activity of the galactoside-specific lectin from mistletoe after tumor destructive therapy in glioma patients." **Anticancer Research** 16:3799–3802, 1996.

65. Lukyanova E.M., Chernyshov V.P., Omelchenko L.J., et al. "Iscador treatment of immuno-compromised children after the Chernobyl accident: clinical and immunological investigations." **Forschende Komplementärmed** 1:58–70, 1994.

66. Luther P. et al. Official report. Forsch Inst Lungenkrankh DDR, Berlin, 1984.

67. Martindale, *The Complete Drug Reference*, Vol. 107, 2001.

68. McNair D., Lorr M., Droppleman L. *Profile of Mood States Manual.* San Diego, CA: EdITS, 1992.

69. Metzner G., Franz H., Kindt A., Fahlbusch B., Suss J. "The *in vitro* activity of lectin I from mistletoe (MLI) and its isolated A and B chains on functions of macrophages and poly-morphonuclear cells." **Immunobiology** 169:461–71, 1985.

70. Metzner G., Franz H., Kindt A., Schumann I., Fahbusch B. "Effects of lectin I from mistletoe (ML-I) and its isolated A and B chains on human mononuclear cells: mitogenic activity and lymphokine release." **Pharmazie** 42(5):337–40, 1988.

71. Mueller E.A., Anderer F.A. "A *Viscum album* oligosaccharide activating human natural cytotoxicity is an interferon gamma inducer." **Cancer Immunol Immunother** 221–227, 1990.

72. Mueller E.A., Anderer F.A. "Chemical specificity of effector cell/tumor cell bridging by a *Viscum album* rhamnogalacturonan enhancing cytotoxicity of human NK cells." **Immunopharmacology** 69–77, 1990.

73. Nail L.M., King K.B. "Fatigue." **Sem Oncol Nurs** 3:257–262, 1987.

74. Neuenschwander, H. & Bruera, E. "Asthenia." In Doyle, D., Hanks, G.W.C., & MacDonald, N. eds. *Oxford Textbook of Palliative Medicine* (2nd Ed.) New York: Oxford University Press. 1998, pp. 573–581.

75. Ovesen L., Allingstrup L., Hannibal J., Mortensen E.L., Hansen O.P. "Effect of dietary counseling on food intake, body weight, response rate, survival, and quality of life in cancer patients undergoing chemotherapy: a prospective, randomized study." **JCO** 11:2043–2049, 1993.

76. Pae H.O.; Seo W.G., Oh G.S., Shin M.K., Lee H.S., Kim S.B., Chung H.T. "Potentiation of tumor necrosis factor-alpha-induced apoptosis by mistletoe lectin." **Immunopharmacol Immunotoxicol** Nov 22(4):697–709, 2000.

77. Pan C.X., et al. "Complementary and alternative medicine in the management of pain, dyspnea, and nausea and vomiting near the end of life: a systematic review." **J Pain Symptom Manage** 20:374–387, 2000.

78. Park R.; Kim M.; So H.; Jung B.; Moon S.; Chung S.; Ko C.; Kim B.; Chung H. "Activation of c-Jun N-terminal kinase 1 (JNK1) in mistletoe lectin II-induced apoptosis of human myeloleukemic U937 cells." **Biochem Pharmacol** Dec 1 60(11):1685–1691, 2000.

79. Reynolds J., (ed). *Martindale Extra Pharmacopoeia.* **AREA?:** Pharmaceutical Press, 1996

80. Ribéreau-Gayon G., Jung M.L., Beck J.P., Anton R. "Effects of serum proteins on the cytotoxic activity and antibody interaction of mistletoe lectins in cell culture." **Planta Med** 59:A673–A674, 1993.

81. Schwabe U., Paffarath D. *Arzneiverordnungsreport 1998.* Heidelberg: Springer Verlag, 1998.

82. Schwartz A.L. "Patterns of Exercise and Fatigue in Physically Active Cancer Survivors." **Oncol Nurs Forum**, April, Volume 25, 1998.

83. Serlin R.C., Mendoza T.R., Nakamura Y., Edwards K.R., Cleeland C.S. "When is cancer pain mild, moderate or severe? Grading pain severity by its interference with function." **Pain** 61:277–284, 1995.

84. Spitzer W.O., Dobson A.J., Hall J., Chesterman E., Levi J., Shepherd R., Battista R.N., Catchlove B.R. "Measuring the quality of life of cancer patients: a concise QL-index for use by physicians." **J Chronic Dis** 34(12):585–97, 1981.

85. Stein G., Berg P.A. "Evaluation of the stimulatory activity of a fermented mistletoe lectin-I free mistletoe extract on T-helper cells and monocytes in healthy individuals in vitro." **Drug Res** 46(6): 35–9, 1996.

86. Stein G.M., Schaller G., Pfüller U., Schietzel M., Büssing A. "Thionins from *Viscum album* L: Influence of the viscotoxins on the activation of granulocytes." **Anticancer Research** 19:1037–1042, 1999.

87. Stirpe F., Legg R.F., Onyon L.J., Ziska P., Franz H. "Inhibition of protein synthesis by a toxic lectin from *Viscum album* L. (mistletoe)." **Biochem J** 190:843-5, 1980.

88. Stumpf C.; Rosenberger A.; Rieger S.; Troger W.; Schietzel M. "Mistletoe extracts in the therapy of malignant, hematological and lymphatic diseases—a monocentric, retrospective analysis over 16 years." **Forsch Komplementarmed Klass Naturheilkd** Jun 7(3):139–46, 2000.

89. "SUPPORT Principle Investigators. Controlled trial to improve care for seriously ill hospitalized patients: Study to understand prognosis and preferences for outcomes and risks for treatment (SUPPORT)." **JAMA**. 274:1591–1598, 1995.

90. Tamburini M., Filiberti A., Barbieri A., Zanoni F., Pizzocaro G., Barletta L., Ventafridda V. "Psychological

aspects of testis cancer therapy: a prospective study." **J Urol** Dec 142(6):1487–9, 1989.

91. Wagner R. "Treatment of Cancer with Iscar: 160 Frequently Asked Questions and Answers." Spring Valley, NY: Mercury Press, 2000, pp. 25–26.

92. Wolf P., Freudenberg N., Konitzer M. "Analgetische und stimmungsaufhellende wirkung bei malignom-patienten unter hochdosierter *Viscum-album*-infusiontherapie." **Erfahrungsheilkunde** 43(5):262–4, 1994.

93. Zhu H.G., Zollner T.M., Klein-Franke A., Anderer F.A. "Activation of human monocyte/macrophage cytotoxicity by IL-2/IFNy is linked to increased expression of an antitumor receptor with specificity for acetylated mannose." **Immunology Letters** 38:111–119, 1993.

Glossary

antihistamine: medication against allergic reactions.

antigen: alien protein that causes the formation of antibodies in the body, which then make the protein harmless.

antibody: defense substance formed as a reaction to the invasion of an *antigen in the blood serum.

antibody formation: an immune reaction.

anti-proliferative effect: acting against proliferative multiplication of tissue.

ascites: abdominal dropsy; collection of fluid in the abdominal cavity.

bradycardia: slow cardiac activity, slow beating of the heart.

cell membrane: forms the cell surface; represents a barrier through which some substances, eg. water, can move through, others eg. sugar, not.

chemotaxis: orientation movement triggered by chemical stimuli.

collum carcinoma: cervical cancer.

colon carcinoma: cancer of the large intestine.

craurosis vulvae: shrinking of the transitional mucous membranes (in this case of the vagina). Also known as Breisky's disease.

cytokine: see lymphokine.

cytotoxic: cell poisoning, cell damaging.

desensitization: artificial reduction of a specific oversensitivity (eg. an allergy); it is possible to test which substance the patient is reacting to; the patient is injected with the smallest quantities that give a hardly discernable reaction, which is increased gradually, to achieve insensitivity.

differential blood count: counting white blood cells with an isochromatic method.

effector: substance that regulates an enzyme reaction.

enteral: regarding the intestine.

enzyme: organic compounds in living cells, which regulates the metabolism of the organism.

eosinophil: white blood cells colored with eosin (a red dye).

erythrocytes: red blood cells.

esophagus: gullet.

granulocytes: a type of white blood cell.

hematopoiesis: blood formation.

Hodgkin's disease: malignant lymph-oma that probably arises from the lymph nodes; malignant disease of the blood.

hypertension: high blood pressure.

hyperthyroidism: overactive thyroid.

immune suppressant: medication that suppresses immune reactions.

immune system: a functional unity including immune cells, other cells and organs, which preserves the individual structures and functions of the organism by working together in the fight against foreign substances; the thymus gland is essential for the immune system, as is the system containing the liver, spleen, lymphatic system and bone marrow.

immune tolerance: the level beyond which an individual does not react normally to an immunogenic stimulus, in other words does not respond to an antigen by forming antibodies.

inoculate: to bring pathogens, tissue, cell material into an organism.

inotropic: influencing the strength or contraction power of the heart muscle; increasing: positively inotropic; reducing: negatively inotropic.

interleukin I: stimulates T and B lymphocytes.

interleukins: signal substances for immune regulation.

intracutaneous: into the skin.

intraperitoneal: into the abdominal cavity.

intubation: insertion of a tube, eg. airway tube through the nose or mouth.

killer cells: sensitized T lymphocytes; excrete cell poisons in the presence of cells containing foreign antigens (eg. transplanted cells, tumor cells).

leukopenia: depleted total leukocyte count.

"Leukotriene"/prostaglandin: prostaglandin.

leukocytes: white blood cells; made up of granulocytes (sixty to seventy percent), lymphocytes (twenty to thirty percent) and monocytes (two to six percent of the blood leukocytes); in infectious illnesses there is a gradual change in the leukocyte division, which can be seen in the differential blood count, and which enables a conclusion to be drawn about the illness.

lymphocytes: white blood cells that originate in the stem cells of bone marrow; formed in the bone marrow, lymph nodes, thymus and spleen, and mostly end up in the blood via the lymphatic system.

lymphokines: substances produced and excreted by the lymphocytes, which activate other cells and influence their function for the

formation of various
enzymes.

macrophages: large *phagocytes

mastopathy: proliferating
nodule and cyst formation,
tissue multipli-cation,
processes of change in the
mammary glands.

metaplasia: curable change of
differentiated tissue into
another type of differentiated tissue.

mitogens: substances that effect
cell division.

mutagen: triggers mutation.

mutation: change, alteration.

neutrophile: easy to color with
chemically neutral sub-
stances, especially susceptible to neutral colorants, eg.
of leukocytes.

non-Hodgkin lymphoma:
malignant lymphoma.

papillomatosis:cauliflower-like
growth.

phagocytes: Cells that are free
in the blood (white blood
cells), and are able to
absorb and to make harm-
less alien substances, especially bacteria, by means of
*enzymes. According to

place of origin, prevalence
and tasks, there are eg. his-
tiocytes, monocytes,
macrophages, microphages.

phagocytosis: dissolving and
making harmless of alien
substances in the organism
by means of phagocytes.

plasma: 1. living substance. 2.
clottable body fluid, eg.
blood plasma, muscle
plasma, albumen contain-
ing liquid gained by press-
ing live muscles.

plasma cell tumor: multiple
myeloma, Kahler's disease;
cancerous swelling in the
bone marrow which origi-
nates from a single, malignant degenerate plasma cell
type (B cell of the immune
system).

plasma expander: plasma sub-
stitute, solutions of natural
or synthetic colloids.

pleura: covering of the lung
tissue.

prospective studies: possibility;
with regard to the future.

prostaglandin: local hormones
that are biologically highly
active and originate from
the different body tissues;

very important for cell function and act as transmitters.

proteins: general description of albumens.

randomization: a selection that allows an exact calculation of random dispersion, based on the probability of theoretical assumptions; serves for the attainment of representability of random checks and experiments.

reactive protein: a protein located in the liver which can attain serum concentrations thousands of times higher than average by means of increased synthesis, in the case of infectious and non-infectious, inflammatory and dying off processes.

receptors: reception devices of the organism for particular stimuli.

resorption: absorption of dissolved substances in the blood and lymphatic system.

reticulo-endothelial: a cell system belonging to the immune system.

system: resorbing inner surface of the body. Especially plays an important role in healing chronic illnesses.

selenium: important trace element; contained in bones and teeth.

subcutaneous: under the skin.

sub-ileus: disturbance of the intestinal movement as early symptom of intestinal obstruction.

suppressor cells: suppress the immune reaction of other, especially T helper cells.

stenocardia: (angina pectoris): heart complaint appearing as labored respiration; due to a functional disturbance of the coronary artery, which supplies the heart muscle with blood.

T helper cells: lymphocytes important for the regulation of immune reactions.

tumor markers: substances traceable in the blood serum that allow conclusions to be drawn about a particular tumor.

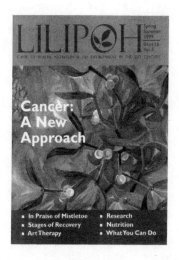